Contents

Preface   **vii**
Acknowledgements   **ix**

Chapter 1   1
Introduction to Cancer

Chapter 2   11
Introduction to Palliative Care

Chapter 3   16
Bereavement and Loss

Chapter 4   25
Ethical Issues in Cancer and Palliative Care

Chapter 5   30
The Multi-professional Team

Chapter 6   34
Communication in Cancer and Palliative Care

Chapter 7   38
The Management of Cancer Pain

Chapter 8   51
Managing Distressing Symptoms

Chapter 9   68
Specialist Palliative Care

Chapter 10   72
Palliative Care Emergencies

Chapter 11   80
Terminal Care

References   87
Appendix   93
Index   105

Preface

This book is not for specialist palliative care nurses. It is for every nurse or health care professional who deals with cancer patients on a daily basis. Basic palliative care is a skill that everyone who cares for this group of patients should possess; that is what this book is about. Both authors have experiences of patients who do not receive the level of palliative and terminal care that should be their right.

Nurses working in acute medical and surgical wards will find this book an excellent introduction to the subject of palliative care in cancer and it should be the first stage introduction to palliative care. There are many palliative care texts which contain detailed information on palliative care and nursing in great depth. This book is not like that; it is intended as a book that you will pick up and thumb frequently when a palliative cancer care patient comes onto the ward. We hope that it will be a useful 'how to' book that will become a friend to the acute care nurse.

George Hogg
Paul Christie

Acknowledgements

We would like to acknowledge the continuing support of both our families through the time we have been working on this book.

We would also like to thank Patricia O'Gorman and the Palliative Care Group at Glasgow Royal Infirmary for their help and permission to use the Palliative Care Guidelines developed after a lot of hard work on their part. Our thanks go, too, for their help and support for the project to Lyndsey Adams and Doreen Donald. And we thank all those friends and colleagues who have taken an interest in the book.

CHAPTER 1

Introduction to Cancer

It is important for nurses caring for people with cancer to have a basic understanding of the causes and management of cancer as a disease. Cancer is a huge health problem and is diagnosed in one in 250 men, and one in 300 women every year (Souhami and Tobias, 1998). In this introductory chapter, the authors look at the epidemiology of cancer, screening and health education, the diagnosis and staging of the disease, and treatment using surgery, radiotherapy and chemotherapy.

Epidemiology of cancer

A number of factors have been associated with the development of cancer but sometimes it is not possible to say for definite why someone develops the disease. Factors identified as causing cancer (carcinogens) are described as *intrinsic* (occurring within the body) or *extrinsic* (occurring outside the body), and have been subdivided as follows:

Intrinsic factors	Genetic susceptibility
	Hormones
Extrinsic factors	Chemicals
	Physical agents (ionising and/or ultraviolet radiation)
	Viruses

Genetic susceptibility

Cellular defects which lead to a change in the genes within the chromosome of a cell have been identified as carcinogenic. Adenomatous polyposis coli (colon cancer) and familial breast cancer are two of those identified as having a genetic cause.

Hormonal causes

This is most commonly seen as a cause of breast cancer, prostate cancer and cancer of the body of the uterus. Hormones are often also used in the treatment of these cancers.

Chemicals

These can be further divided into three groups: (1) occupational chemicals, (2) environmental chemicals and (3) social chemicals.

1. Occupational chemicals – have been identified as asbestos, arsenic, benzene, chromium, nickel and petroleum fractions (oil) (Goyns, Hancock and Rees, 1996). These chemicals are direct causes of lung cancer, mesothelioma and cancers of the head and neck.
2. Environmental chemicals – these are usually related to dietary intake and have been identified as causing colorectal and oesophageal cancers. Preservatives and food colourings are also implicated.
3. Social chemicals – such as smoking and alcohol are implicated in causing lung cancer, cancers of the head and neck, oesophageal and gastric cancer.

Radiation

Ionising radiation causes changes in the molecular structure of living cells and leads to damage of molecular DNA. Some of these changes lead to cell death, but less severe changes change the cells' control mechanism and they become neoplastic. Radiation is implicated in skin cancer, lung cancer, bone tumours, thyroid cancer and leukaemia.

Viruses

This is less certain (Carter and Neville, 1988) but viruses such as hepatitis B have been implicated in liver cancer and human papilloma virus in cervical cancer.

Screening

The aim of cancer screening is to detect the disease at an early stage and thereby improve the possible cure rate. Screening is now well established in breast cancer (mammography) and in cervical cancer (smear tests). Both of these programmes have shown benefits, with early detection and treatment shown to improve survival from these diseases (Tabar et al, 1992, Lindbrick et al, 1996).

Screening for colorectal cancer using faecal occult blood testing (FOBT) and sigmoidoscopy has not been proven to increase cure rates (Hardcastle et al, 1989; Kirby et al, 1998). At the present time a study is under way in the United Kingdom to examine the consequences of a national screening programme. It is also possible to screen for prostate cancer using a blood test to measure the levels of prostate specific antigen (PSA). However, this has not been widely introduced due to the difficulties in setting up and maintaining a widespread screening programme, e.g. should all men above a certain age be screened, should only those with a family history be included?.

Routine cancer screening also has disadvantages. It can lead to increased anxiety in both individuals and the population as a whole. Telling 'healthy' people that they might have a life-threatening disease needs a lot of care and attention to the psychological implications. There are also huge implications for the widespread implementation of screening programmes which will no doubt occupy scientists, clinicians and politicians for a long time to come.

Health education

Most of us fear the word cancer and much of the population still see it as an incurable disease. Nearly everyone has known someone who has died of cancer. It has to be said that some forms of the disease are curable if caught at an early stage and treated. Most people, however, still present for treatment too late and there are a number of reasons for this. Ignorance, misconception and embarrassment are common (Lorigan and Hancock, 1996).

The media have an important role to play and health education is a major component of the remit of all health boards and authorities. Tobacco is a major health education issue.

However, despite health education and screening cancer still affects many people. Once the disease has been suspected what is the next stage in the patient's journey?

Diagnosis and staging of cancer

The treatment of cancer is often unpleasant, with profound effects on the patient's and family's physical and psychosocial well-being. The diagnosis of cancer instills fear and dread in most people. Like all other diseases an accurate diagnosis is the first step in devising a treatment plan. Some of the common investigations used at this stage are:

1. *Tissue biopsy* – this involves the microscopic examination of suspect tissue. The samples can be obtained by needle biopsy where a fine needle is used to aspirate some cells under local anaesthetic. Incision biopsy using a scalpel to remove a small piece of the tumour, again under local anaesthetic, or an *en bloc* dissection of the tumour under general anaesthesia may also be used (see 'Cancer surgery', below).

2. *Blood samples* – a full blood count is essential. Specific reference is made to the erythrocyte sedimentation rate (ESR), and red and white cell counts. Biochemical tests of liver function, urea and electrolytes are also routine.

3. *Radiological investigations* – plain X-rays of the chest can show metastases in the lung and often preclude further more expensive investigations. Barium swallow and enema investigations will show gastrointestinal cancers. Ultrasound is becoming increasingly common because it is simple, cheap, non-invasive and accurate. Its main use in oncology is in the diagnosis of abdominal masses, liver and lymph node metastases and the detection of hydronephrosis (a common complication of some cancers). Complex investigations such as computerised tomography (CT) and magnetic resonance imaging (MRI) are often reserved for the detection of tumours not revealed by other methods.

4. *Nuclear medicine scans* – in these investigations a radioisotope is given either by mouth or by intravenous injection to the patient. Measurements of the uptake of the isotope into certain tissues are then made using a gamma camera. The main uses are in bone scanning, where lesions show up as increased uptake (hot spots), usually indicating bone metastases, and in thyroid cancer, where a reduced uptake (cold spots) indicates a neoplasm. Lung scans are used to identify pulmonary emboli, another common complication of cancer.

5. *History and examination* – a full physical examination of the patient is vital. The patient is asked about any abnormal findings they have noticed, such as a lump, changes in bowel or bladder habits, abnormal bleeding, pain or weight loss. The doctor will record the size, shape, position and mobility of any lumps detected. An examination of the regional lymph nodes is made to detect any metastatic spread. The liver is palpated as well as the abdomen.

Staging

Before a treatment plan can be devised for the patient the extent of the disease has to be known. This is called staging and has the following purposes:

- preparation of an individual treatment plan;
- estimating prognosis;
- comparing similar cases and treatment trials;
- accurate documentation;
- understanding tumour biology.

The recognised method of staging tumours is now the TNM system developed by the American Joint Committee on Cancer Staging and End Result Reporting (International Union Against Cancer, 1997). In this system T relates to the size of the primary tumour, N to the absence or presence and extent of regional lymph node metastases, and M to the absence or presence of distant metastases. Staging gives an insight to the likely outcome of treatment and life expectancy.

Staging can be pathological – surgical specimen, biopsy; clinical – from examination; or non-clinical – from blood tests, or X-rays (Neal and Hoskin, 1997).

Treatment

Once the diagnosis has been made, the next stage is to devise a treatment plan for the patient. With cancer this is based on a number of factors and three levels of decision-making have been identified (Neal and Hoskin, 1997):

1. The decision to treat or not to treat.
2. Treatment intent, radical or palliative.
3. Specific aspects of treatment policy regarding local, systemic and supportive therapy (Figure 1.1).

Radical treatment is given with the intent to cure or control the disease long term. Palliative treatment is given to improve the patient's quality of life or control symptoms. It will not improve their survival. As Figure 1.1 shows, treatment tends to involve surgery, radiotherapy, chemotherapy, or a combination of them all. We now look at these treatment methods in a little more detail.

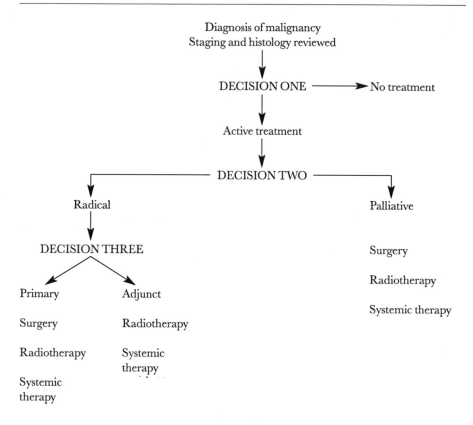

Figure 1.1. Treatment options. (Source: Neal and Hoskin, 1997.)

Cancer surgery

This is the oldest and most common treatment for cancer (James, 1991). Table 1.1 shows some of the 'landmarks' noted in cancer surgery (Raven, 1984).

The aim of cancer surgery was to cure the patient. It was thought that removing the tumour as a whole (*en bloc*) and dissecting out the regional lymph nodes would prevent tumour spread and effect a cure. This was not the case unfortunately and approximately 70% of patients were found to have microscopic distant metastases (Rosenberg, 1985). Research into the nature of tumours, growth and spread has led to the realisation that surgery alone is not able to cure disease that has already metastasised to other sites.

Surgery does, however, have an important part to play in cancer treatment, and can be curative in certain cases, e.g. thyroid cancer and skin cancer.

Table 1.1. Landmarks in cancer surgery

Surgeon	Year	Operation
Billroth	1881	Subtotal gastrectomy
Halsted	1890	Radical mastectomy
Schlatter	1897	Total gastrectomy
Mikulicz	1898	Oesophagogastrectomy
Wertheim	1900	Radical hysterectomy
Miles	1908	Abdominoperineal excision of rectum
Tarek	1913	Oesophagectomy
Trotter	1913	Partial pharyngectomy
Graham and Singer	1933	Pneumonectomy

However, today it is used in conjunction with radiotherapy and chemotherapy in what is known as adjunct therapy. It also has a part to play in the diagnosis and staging of cancer, as stated earlier. Testicular tumours are treated and staged by orchidectomy and it is now usual for breast lumps to be removed at lumpectomy rather than mastectomy.

Later in the course of the disease patients might require palliative surgery to help relieve distressing symptoms such as the removal of single lung or liver metastasis, oophorectomy to effect hormonal manipulation or laminectomy in spinal cord compression. Surgeons might also be involved in the insertion of skin-tunnelled central venous catheters for the administration of cytotoxic chemotherapy.

Radiotherapy

The use of ionising radiation as a cytotoxic agent is known as radiotherapy. With the discovery of X-rays by William Roentgen and isolation of radium by Pierre and Marie Curie, at the end of the nineteenth century, came the hope that radiation would be the miracle cure for most ills (Snape and Robinson, 1988). However, as Marie Curie and other pioneers of radioactivity found to their cost, radiation has dangers. It is a fine line between the treatment effect and the side effects, which makes modern radiotherapy very complex. In a chapter of this size, we can give only a brief outline of this cancer treatment method. However, a basic understanding of radiotherapy treatment will allow the nurse to understand better what patients experience as part of their cancer treatment.

Radiotherapy works at cellular level by causing damage to the double helix strand of DNA. This causes disruption inside the cell and when it comes to divide, it cannot. This means that tumour growth is stopped.

Normal cells are also affected but their chances of repair and growth are better, allowing quicker recovery from the effects of radiation.

X-rays are the most common type of radiation in use today. They are produced and delivered by machines called linear accelerators which deliver a concentrated beam of radiation. This method is known as teletherapy and careful planning is required to ensure a therapeutic dose is given with minimal side effects to the patient. This is carried out by a consultant radiotherapist (doctor), in conjunction with therapy radiographers, who carry out the treatment. In some cases such as head and neck tumours, where damage to vital structures can occur from small doses of radiation, an immobilising shell has to be made. This is a detailed and important part of the planning and needs time.

Radiotherapy is given in doses known as fractions, usually five times a week (Monday–Friday) for a period of 3–6 weeks, if the treatment is radical. Between one and five treatments are given for palliative therapy, but this depends on the consultant carrying out the planning. Many patients attend as out-patients as the treatment itself only takes a few minutes. Whilst the machine is switched on it is producing radiation; therefore the patient is alone in the treatment room being observed by the radiographer on camera.

There are side effects to external beam radiotherapy, which is seen as a local therapy in that it focuses on the tumour site. The first of these is possible skin reactions at the beam entry and exit site. Patients are given careful explanations about skin care and what to do if a reaction does occur, and it is important that they follow these guidelines to prevent further damage.

Systemic side effects include fatigue/weakness which usually increases as the treatment progresses. Nausea can be a problem, especially when the abdomen or oesophagus is being treated. Bone marrow depression can also occur if the pelvis, spine, ribs, sternum and skull are within the treatment zone. In this case a full blood count should be taken weekly. Other common problems are mucositis and alopecia if the head and neck are being treated. It is important for nurses looking after radiotherapy patients to be aware of these side effects.

As well as external beam radiotherapy, some cancers such as those of the cervix or uterus can be treated using internal radiation or brachytherapy. This is very specialised treatment and is only carried out in specialist oncology units under strict control. It is done on an in-patient basis, with the patient isolated in a special suite for 24–48 hours. Careful planning, patient preparation and ongoing care are required when brachytherapy is used.

Radiotherapy, like most cancer treatments, is a team effort and involves oncologists, radiographers, physicists, technicians and nurses. The aim is to ensure that the patient receives the optimal care.

Chemotherapy

The use of cytotoxic drugs in cancer treatment is known as a systemic therapy. Whilst the effects of radiotherapy are directed at the tumour site, chemotherapy affects the whole body via the bloodstream. Most chemotherapy agents are given intravenously or via a central venous catheter.

Like radiotherapy, chemotherapy agents act in the cell and can be described as *cycle specific* or *phase specific*. Cycle specific drugs can be further classified as alkylating agents, and phase specific drugs as antimetabolites.

1. Alkylating agents – react with and bind together DNA, preventing cell division. Examples are platinum and cyclophosphamide.
2. Antimetabolites – prevent the formation of nucleic acid and interfere with DNA/RNA synthesis, thus causing cell death. Examples are methotrexate and 5-fluorouracil (5-FU).
3. Anti-tumour antibiotics – act similarly to alkylating agents and antimetabolites. Examples are mitomycin and bleomycin.
4. Plant-derived cytotoxics – the action of these agents is more complex, but their use is increasing. Examples are vincristine, etoposide and paclitaxol.

Like radiotherapy, chemotherapy is usually given in a specialist oncology unit. However, patients who are being given chemotherapy may be admitted to general surgical or medical wards for many other reasons. Therefore an understanding of the basics of treatment and the side effects is important.

Side effects of chemotherapy

1. Nausea and vomiting – these are often cited as the most distressing side effects of chemotherapy (Coates et al, 1983). Prophylactic anti-emetics are the treatment of choice. It is also important to maintain an adequate fluid and diet intake. Other supportive care includes teaching relaxation techniques.
2. Mouth problems – such as dryness, altered taste, or mucositis are common. Good oral hygiene and regular nursing assessment are

imperative. Chlorhexidine (Corsodyl) and benzydamine (Difflam) are commonly used mouthwashes for such cases.

3. Diarrhoea – is usually controlled with loperamide or codeine phosphate.

4. Nephrotoxicity – damage to the kidneys is a problem with some drugs and accurate fluid balance and intake are vital parts of the treatment regime. Regular blood biochemistry is also carried out.

5. Peripheral neuropathy – 'pins and needles' in the fingers and toes can occur with vincristine and cisplatin. Assessment of the patient, and reporting such symptoms to medical staff, will often lead to a dose reduction or cessation of use of the agent concerned.

6. Alopecia – this is often one of the most distressing symptoms, especially in women. Pre-treatment referral for a wig is important. Counselling and advice about using mild shampoos, avoiding perms and dyeing are important as well.

CHAPTER 2

Introduction to Palliative Care

Although huge advances are being made in understanding of the causes and nature of cancer, cure rates for many forms of the disease have not improved significantly for many years. Until fairly recently palliation was the only treatment available for many cancers. The importance of effective palliation therefore cannot be overstated. This chapter gives nurses an introduction to palliative care as a concept, and the different forms it can take.

The development of palliative care

The first hospice for the care of the dying was probably established in France in 1842 and the movement quickly spread to Ireland and the United Kingdom. Although many of these hospices were built to care for those with advanced tuberculosis, one founded in County Cork was specifically for cancer. Mostly founded and run by Catholic Orders, the hospices were not part of mainstream health care. The physicians, priests and nuns who staffed the institutions focused on spirituality, and social and psychological care of the residents. As in modern hospices, lay carers and volunteers had a big part to play in the care of sufferers.

During the 1940s the biomedical model of care come into vogue. The first cytotoxic drugs were being discovered and their clinical application to cancer treatment was realised (Coleman and Hancock, 1996). The use of cytotoxic chemotherapy flourished during the 1950s and 1960s, when many expected these drugs to provide a miracle cure for cancer. Unfortunately this was not to be (Woodruff, 1999). This reliance on science and cure at all costs (the horrendous side effects of chemotherapy were seen as a necessary evil) developed into a lack of attention to the patient as a person by many medical staff. Disease-orientated medicine was becoming normal practice.

The modern hospice movement

It was during her training as a nurse, social worker, and ultimately a doctor that Dame Cicely Saunders developed an interest in the care of the dying. Throughout her previous careers and during her medical school training, Saunders was aware of the distress being caused to those with incurable disease. She went to work at St Lukes Home for the Dying Poor in London, where she learned about the use of regular oral morphine in cancer pain. It was here that she worked closely with its founder, Dr Howard Barrett, and in 1967 she left to set up St Christopher's Hospice in Sydenham, London.

At St Christopher's care was provided to those with advanced cancer which focused on the psychological, social, spiritual, holistic management of patients and their families. Saunders ensured that there was a major educational and research commitment, and encouraged multidisciplinary teamwork. This would ensure that the work being done could be seen alongside the traditional scientific and clinical care being delivered in hospitals, thus validating what was being done in the eyes of her peers in the medical profession.

Although the number of hospices continued to grow during the 1970s and 1980s, a number of studies (Cartwright et al, 1973; Lunt and Hillier, 1981; Bowling, 1983; Herd, 1990) demonstrated that most people were still dying in acute and general hospitals. It has since been identified that whilst one-third of terminally ill patients will die within a week of their final admission to hospital, 40% will stay in hospital for more than a month (Wilkes, 1984). The discharge rate for terminally ill patients is higher in teaching hospitals than in district general hospitals, and patients who die tend to be younger – 50% are under 65 compared with 30% in district general hospitals (Cartwright et al, 1973).

In light of this, many teaching and acute hospitals now have hospital palliative care teams (HPCT), who offer support and advice on the care of patients with advanced cancer. Very often these teams have close links with the local hospice or National Health Service Palliative Care Unit. This means that those suitable for hospice care can be referred at an appropriate stage in their illness to benefit fully from the type of care given in such units (Wilkes, 1980).

The definition and goals of palliative care

The generally accepted definition of palliative care is that devised by the World Health Organization (WHO, 1990):

> Palliative care is the active, total care of patients whose disease is not responsive to cura-
> tive treatment. Control of pain, of other symptoms and of psychological, social and spir-
> itual problems is paramount. The goal of palliative care is the achievement of the best
> quality of life for patients and their families. Many aspects of palliative care are also
> applicable earlier in the course of the illness, in conjunction with anti cancer treatment.

It is vital for nurses working with cancer patients to be aware of the holistic nature of palliative care, and to know that effective palliative care can
be given in any health care location.

In 1995 the National Council for Hospice and Specialist Palliative
Care Services (NCHSPCS) aimed to clarify the different levels of pallia-
tive care that could be provided to patients. This work was based on the
WHO definition and led to the following definitions:

1. Basic palliative care – care delivery with a palliative approach is a core
   skill which every health professional in whatever setting should possess
   if dealing with patients with an incurable, progressive disease.
2. Specialised palliative interventions – are non-curative treatments
   aimed specifically at modifying the illness. They are performed by
   specialists in clinical, medical oncology, or surgery.
3. Specialist palliative care – is care delivered by a multidisciplinary team
   led by clinicians with recognised specialist palliative medicine training.
   The team works in collaboration with those providing a palliative
   approach and deals with the more complex problems to ensure that
   patient and family needs are met.

Basic palliative care and specialist palliative care tend to be based on the
hospice model of care, focusing on psychosocial and spiritual needs as
well as physical care. Specialised palliative interventions tend to focus on
the biomedical model of care, which is disease oriented and prevalent in
acute and oncology settings. It is with this in mind that this book will
focus on the *palliative approach*, ensuring that readers have a grounding in
this method of care.

The palliative approach has as its main priority the promotion of physical, psychological and spiritual well-being of the patient and family. By
focusing on quality of life, best possible symptom control and a quality death
in an holistic manner, the nursing management of patients is enhanced.

The need for palliative care

Within a population of 1 000 000 people, approximately 2800 will die
from cancer, 2400 of them will have pain, 1300 breathing difficulties and
1400 nausea or vomiting (Higginson, 1997). As we said previously, many

of these people will die in hospital under the care of medical, surgical and oncology nurses; therefore an understanding of the concepts of the palliative approach is vital.

Whilst this book focuses on palliative care in cancer, nurses should note that the palliative approach is becoming increasingly important in other life-threatening diseases.

The chapters on communication, symptom control, loss and bereavement, and terminal care are therefore relevant to many areas. Higginson (1993) states:

> The concept of palliative care has broadened over time from 'terminal care' to include the care of those who have life threatening disease but are not imminently dying. Including people who have recently been diagnosed with advanced cancer and those who have other life threatening diseases such as multiple sclerosis, motor neurone disease, AIDS, chronic circulatory or respiratory disease.

Twycross (1999) identifies three essential components of palliative care and states that any activity in one area will impact on the others (Figure 2.1).

Teamwork and partnership means that we work with the patient, family and other professionals to ensure that appropriate, effective care is delivered. It is unlikely that this will be an equal partnership as the roles and responsibilities of the team will differ greatly (see Chapter 5). This recognition of the elements of good teamwork is one of the achievements of palliative care.

Psychosocial support is key to the provision of palliative care and is prevalent throughout literature and practice.

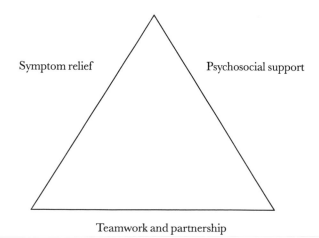

Figure 2.1. Three essential components of palliative care.

The NCHSPCS (1997a) say 'Psychosocial care is concerned with the psychological and emotional well being of the patient and their family/carers, including issues of self-esteem, insight into and adaptation to the illness and its consequences, communication, social functioning and relationships'. Psychosocial support is very much a dimension of the various disciplines involved in palliative care.

Symptom relief is often seen as the biggest chunk of palliative care; indeed the word palliative derives from the Latin 'to cloak' which relates to the cloaking of symptoms of disease. Table 2.1 gives an indication of the type and prevalence of various symptoms that readers might encounter. Generally symptoms can be caused by:

- cancer;
- treatment regimes;
- other pathology.

Once again the crossover to psychosocial support and teamwork features in that we often need to involve specialists to deal with certain symptoms, and explanations and support are always vital. Many symptoms are made worse by fear, worry or depression (Finlay, 1995).

Whilst this chapter has given a very brief introduction to palliative care those that follow will build on this, leading to a greater understanding.

Table 2.1. Symptoms experienced by cancer patients

Symptom	Bruera et al (1991)[a] (n = 275)	Hockley et al (1998)[b] (n = 26)
	Incidence (%)	
Weakness/Fatigue	90	88
Anorexia	85	92
Pain	76	69
Nausea	68	54
Constipation	65	54
Sedation/Confusion	60	34
Dyspnoea	12	69
Insomnia		88
Sore mouth		81
Pressure sores		61[c]

[a]Cancer patients only.
[b]Patients referred from Respiratory Directorate (cancer and non-malignant disease).
[c]Worse in patients with non-malignancies.
From Dunlop and Hockley (1998).

CHAPTER 3

Bereavement and Loss

In this chapter the authors look at the concepts of bereavement and loss as they relate to the diagnosis and treatment of cancer, although many of the concepts apply equally to the diagnosis and management of any life-threatening illness.

Everyone has experienced a loss at some point in their lives, whether it was the loss of a favourite toy as a child, the loss of a family pet, changes in relationships as we grow older. Whilst we learn to cope with these 'mini-mal' losses, nothing can prepare us to cope with the loss of a loved one whether they be family, partner or friend (Kendrick, 1998).

An understanding of the concept of loss and its consequences for those left behind is important when caring for patients and their families experiencing cancer and palliative care. The psychosocial effects of a major loss through bereavement are now well documented. In his study Jacobs (1993) found that up to one-third of those affected by the death of a spouse or child will have a physical or mental health problem. Clegg (1988) notes that 31% of elderly patients in an acute psychiatric unit had been recently bereaved. Therefore it can be seen that loss is a common, and often unrecognised, cause of illness. Archer (1991) states 'There are many reasons for health professionals to understand the process of grief'. Bereavement is a time of great vulnerability and stress for most people, and is usually accompanied by a certain degree of deterioration in physical health and psychosocial well-being. Nurses often play a pivotal role in helping people to cope with loss of varying degrees; however, when it comes to loss through life-threatening illness we often feel ill equipped to cope. This chapter will give nurses a better understanding of how much they can do.

The diagnosis of cancer

When given a diagnosis of 'cancer' most people react in the same way. Very often they will say, 'You must be wrong' 'Are you sure it's me?'

Kubler-Ross (1970) talks about this 'Denial Stage' in her work, which we will look at in some detail later. She found that nearly half of those questioned gave similar, if not the same, response when diagnosed. As well as this psychological reaction many people have physical symptoms. These were described by Worden (1982) as:

- experience of hollowness in the abdomen and tightness in the throat;
- oversensitivity to noise;
- a sense of depersonalisation – nothing feels real;
- breathlessness associated with deep, sighing respiration;
- muscular weakness;
- lack of energy and fatigue;
- dry mouth.

Such a diagnosis will also impact on the family and they too can suffer the same symptoms. Therefore nurses who are likely to be with patients when this news is given, or deal with the patient in the immediate aftermath, should be aware of the effects. Psychological support is vital during this period; therefore this will be examined more closely in this chapter.

The psychological impact of cancer

We have already said that cancer and its management can cause untold stress, yet it is only fairly recently that the true psychological impact has been investigated (Moorey, 1992). In a study of patients in a Canadian Oncology Clinic, Farber et al (1984) reported that 34% of the patients had 'high and clinically significant levels of psychological distress'. The close family of patients must also be considered at this stage as many similar studies have shown that they too are victims. Coursey et al (1975) found that stress levels are often higher in the immediate family than in the patients themselves. It is important therefore for nurses to realise this and understand why some people will act they way they do to cope with the news and their future.

Lazarus and Folkman (1984) suggested a three-stage model for coping with the stress of cancer, thus:

1. Primary appraisal – is there a threat?
2. Secondary appraisal – what can be done about it?
3. Coping – implementing strategies for coping.

Primary appraisal

At this stage the patient and family need to come to terms with the diagnosis and decide how life-threatening the illness is. How they do this will depend very much on what they are told at diagnosis, and how they are told. How many of us have been present when the consultant or registrar stands at the bottom of the patient's bed during the ward round and tells the patient in an off the cuff manner that they have cancer and there is nothing that can be done? This inability of doctors to break bad news appropriately has been recognised, is being addressed by the profession and will be looked at in the next chapter.

If the cancer has been identified at an early stage and the patient is being offered 'curative' treatment, then this will give them more hope than if they are told that the disease is advanced and management will be 'palliative'. The majority of people, however, will still react in the same way at this stage and view the diagnosis as a 'death sentence' (Greer, 1985). Often with more information about treatment modalities, nursing care etc. (see Chapter 1), the patient and family will move on to stage two.

Secondary appraisal

This is when detailed information and talk of the future come in. The patient should be given explanations about possible treatment plans and the effects they might have (see Chapter 1). Most people will know of someone who has had cancer and many will have horror stories to tell about hair loss, nausea, vomiting, weight loss etc. At this stage it is often desirable for the patient and family to be in contact with someone other than the person who gave them the diagnosis. It is a common reaction to 'blame' the person breaking the bad news, and this often affects how they perceive any information given by that person in the future (Buckman, 1984). In times gone by the bearer of bad news was often killed after giving it (Kaye, 1996)! At this stage it is common for the family to be introduced to a Macmillan nurse (see Chapter 5), for detailed information, support and counselling. The patient and family need time to assimilate this information and very often will ask the ward nurse to reinforce what was said.

Coping

It is during this stage of adjustment that most people experience a wide range of emotions – numbness, disbelief, anger, protest, fear, hope and despair (Peck, 1972; Horowitz, 1979; Parkes, 1988). It is not only the patient who is running this gamut of emotions; the family may also be experiencing the same if not stronger feelings. Often, the patient's partner represses their own feelings in order to support the patient (Moorey, 1992). As the patient is very often still in the acute surgical ward at this stage, it is important that nurses do not take the mood swings and emotional outbursts as a personal attack, but realise that they are part of a normal reaction to an extremely abnormal situation. They should also be aware of the roles of other professionals at this difficult time and know when to involve them; this information is given in Chapter 5 of this book.

The social impact of cancer

It is a common reaction for the person diagnosed with cancer to withdraw from normal social contact and activities. People will assume what is described as the 'sick role' (Parsons, 1992), and will give up their independence in the hope that it will help them find help from others (Pugsley and Pardoe, 1992). This will often manifest itself in hospital patients as listlessness, lethargy and helplessness. Such patients can be difficult for nurses to manage alone; therefore recourse to the appropriate team member is advised.

Models of loss and bereavement

A model is something that is not real, but matches or represents reality as closely as possible (Pearson, Vaughan and Fitzgerald, 1996). Models of loss give us a framework of how people might react to life-threatening illness and bereavement, therefore allowing a better understanding of why people act the way they do.

In this chapter we will look at two models. The first was proposed by Elisabeth Kubler-Ross (1970), and the second by Colin Murray Parkes (1972). Although both were developed in the 1970s, they are still seen as major, relevant works by psychologists and sociologists.

Elisabeth Kubler-Ross

Elisabeth Kubler-Ross is an American psychiatrist whose work was carried out in the early 1970s at Chicago University Hospital. She was one of a number of doctors who were becoming increasingly concerned about the shift in medicine towards focusing on the illness and its symptoms rather than the effects it was having on the individual and their family's needs. This led her to think that there was a feeling that death and dying were being ignored or avoided. Especially worrying for her was the growing movement in medicine. She soon realised that although terminally ill patients received excellent nursing and physical care, their emotional, spiritual and psychological needs were not being met as well as they might. She decided to organise a seminar at the University of Chicago to consider the implications of terminal illness for the patient and his/her carer. She invited some patients and carers along to give their account of the illness to a group of medical, sociology, psychology and theology students. The seminar was voted a success and so in future events she invited hospital staff, relatives and friends of the patients to attend.

This meant that having listened to patients and heard what their fears and experiences were, hospital staff became able to respond constructively and effectively to their needs. The patients also found that they were more able to move towards acceptance and peace of mind in relation to their impending death.

Dr Kubler-Ross built on this early work and went on to research the subject in greater depth. This led to her publishing her Stage Model of Loss, which has been expanded and built on since. She proposed that there were five stages that we go through to come to terms with a loss (through bereavement):

1. Denial and isolation.
2. Anger.
3. Bargaining.
4. Depression.
5. Acceptance.

The first version of the model placed people neatly into each stage, one after the other, suggesting that everyone moved through stages 1 to 5 as a natural progression. Further work by both Kubler-Ross and Murray Parkes showed that this is not always the case. People can experience some or all of the stages described at varying times, and for varying lengths of time. In some cases of complex grief, the individual might never accept the loss.

Stage 1: Denial and isolation

As we discovered at the beginning of this chapter, most people will react in the same way to being told that they have a life-threatening illness. The most common response is to suggest to the bearer of the bad news that they have made a mistake.

This initial denial is usually temporary and is very often replaced by partial acceptance of the situation they find themselves in. Kubler-Ross states that it is rare for anyone to continue in denial throughout their illness and goes on to say that of the two hundred patients involved in her study only three attempted to deny death until the very last. Some people's denial can be so strong that they isolate themselves. They refuse to talk to anyone for fear that the subject will be raised. Many will go out of their way to emphasise how good they are feeling and how good their life is in the hope that someone will reassure them and confirm this. When this stage of denial and isolation fails to fulfil their needs many move on to the stage of anger.

Stage 2: Anger

This is one of the most difficult stages for those around the patient to cope with, possibly because the expressions of anger tend to be sporadic and indiscriminate. If the patient is in hospital at this stage the anger tends to be directed at nursing staff. How often have we heard that 'Nothing they do is right', 'They're always too busy with other things to worry about me'. The patient's family and friends often suffer as well, with the anger being vented on them: 'Where have you been, you're late.' Very often the closest family or partner become tearful and upset at this behaviour and can avoid visiting, thus forming a vicious circle of more anger.

Anger is also very often a reaction to the loss of control many people experience as a result of the illness and treatment. The cancer seems to be the controlling influence in the patient's life. Hospital appointments become the 'norm' with allotted times for the doctor, tests, treatment etc.

All of this becomes the main focus of life for both the patient and family, and most of it is beyond their control.

Stage 3: Bargaining

Kubler-Ross states that the stage of bargaining is useful to the patient for short periods of time only. Rather than lose one's temper over the timing of appointments, which tends to go nowhere, the patient will try and negotiate timings, put off treatment for a day or avoid seeing the doctor. This bargaining gives the patient back some control over his life and very often is a chance to be free of the distressing symptoms of the disease and its treatment.

Stage 4: Depression

The stage eventually comes when the patient can no longer deny the existence of the disease. Once surgery, chemotherapy or radiotherapy have taken their toll on his physical being, his hair loss, weight loss and fatigue have taken their toll on his psychosocial being. This is very often when the sense of loss is at its greatest.

As periods of hospitalisation increase the financial burdens become greater. Normal family life is replaced by hospital visiting times, very often with limited privacy.

Many health care professionals are unaware that this is a very important stage in the preparatory grief that terminally ill patients must go through to prepare them for the final separation. Therefore it is vital for patients to have as much contact with their close family and friends as possible. Thus open visiting should be encouraged whenever possible, even in a 'busy' acute ward.

The reaction of many carers at this stage is to try and make the patient 'look on the bright side' and jolly them along. This is very often an expression of our inability to cope with depression. This shows us that there is a need to involve other specialists from the palliative care team with the patient, for example the psychologist or chaplain.

Stage 5: Acceptance

Given time, support and care, most patients eventually come to accept what is wrong with them and what is going to happen. We should not assume that the patient who has accepted is happy after his depression; on the contrary this stage is very often void of any feelings at all. One patient in the Kubler-Ross study described this as 'the final rest before the long journey'.

Colin Murray Parkes

Whilst Elisabeth Kubler-Ross describes five stages through which each patient must pass to come to terms with loss, Colin Murray Parkes (1972) lists four. He is keen to caution people against looking at this as a 'fixed sequence through which every bereaved person must pass in order to recover from bereavement'.

Colin Murray Parkes is honorary consultant psychiatrist to St Christopher's Hospice in London, and consultant psychiatrist to St Joseph's Hospice, also in London. He has lectured widely both in the UK and abroad and is recognised as an expert on bereavement and loss. His Process Model (1972) is probably the most useful tool for nurses working with cancer patients in the acute setting. The model has four phases:

1. Shock, numbness and the pain of grieving.
2. Manifestations of fear, guilt, anger and resentment.
3. Disengagement, apathy and aimlessness.
4. Gradual hope and a move in new directions.

Phase 1: Shock, numbness and the pain of grieving

When we suffer a loss, or are given bad news, we very often find it hard to take in the full reality of the situation. This is especially so if the loss is sudden or unexpected. Parkes says that this feeling of numbness and unreality is almost universal and can last from a few hours to days. It is during this period that people tend to pine for what is being lost, very often crying, making it difficult for others to deal with. Within most Western cultures, crying in public is frowned upon, so patients tend to become isolated and shun company during this period.

Phase 2: Manifestations of fear, guilt, anger and resentment

The majority of us must admit that we have a fear of cancer and dying in pain as a result of the disease. The fear of distressing side effects of treatment, of pain and generally not knowing what is ahead is almost universal. Many patients experience feelings of guilt about what might have been; e.g. 'I should have stopped smoking a long time ago'. Anger tends to be directed at medical and nursing staff: 'Why me, what have I done that's so bad?' Very often the hospital chaplain or the patient's own minister will be of help at this stage. It is important to realise that any feelings directed at you as a nurse are not personal.

Phase 3: Disengagement, apathy and aimlessness

Once the second phase has run its course, everyone has recovered from the gamut of emotions and hopefully come through the other side unscathed. The patient appears to have 'burnt out'. They seem to have lost the fight and urge to go on.

This phase very often comes during the patient's treatment and so is often masked by the physical and mental effects of treatment, although it can manifest itself in acute wards whilst the patient is awaiting treatment, or is not able to receive active treatment due to the extent of disease. This phase is again one that many find difficult to cope with, so it may be advisable to involve specialist colleagues such as a psychologist or counsellor. This phase can last for varying times and can recur during the patient's journey.

Phase 4: Gradual hope and a move in new directions

The one thing that usually persists through all stages of this often long and tortuous journey is hope. Hope that there has been a mistaken diagnosis, hope that research will find a cure, hope that the treatment side effects will be minimal, hope that death will be peaceful and quick. It is vital that those around the patients never relieve the patients of this hope. This can be difficult when we watch patients fight long and hard before succumbing to a frightening or painful death, or we see fit young people go through the indignities of the disease that is cancer, i.e. hair loss, weight loss, only to die prematurely.

Hope is the one weapon we all have, and it should never be taken for granted. Most people will eventually come to terms with or learn to cope with their illness, loss and future. What we as carers need to realise is that the patient's family and friends will have to go through the whole cycle again when the patient does die.

CHAPTER 4

Ethical Issues in Cancer and Palliative Care

This is a difficult subject for any nurse caring for cancer and palliative care patients. However, it is often more difficult for those working outside specialist palliative care units. This chapter therefore introduces the reader to some of the more common ethical problems with which nurses in acute areas might be faced. Ethics is a huge subject in which there are no right or wrong answers, and this chapter provides only an introduction.

Refusing treatment

Under United Kingdom law patients who are conscious and lucid and refuse treatment must have their wishes respected. This is quite clear, but many people will continue to go through distressing and time-consuming hospital treatment in the hope that it will lead to a cure. Whilst no one can give hard and fast claims about how treatment will work, many of us have seen cases where the patient is suffering horrendous side effects from drugs or other treatments. We can see that the patient is not getting better, but believe that it is not our place as nurses to question the management being advocated by a consultant. This is where we need to rely on our own communication skills and experience to be able to advocate for the patient/family, and help them express their feelings on the matter. So long as the family are acting in the best interests of the patient they remain within the law.

Nurses are very often the carer most close to patients and their family. Keeping the patient and family informed at all levels will help when the subject of refusing treatment comes to the fore. The problem is very often that the physician knows that he or she is overtreating the patient but does not know how or when to stop (Solomon et al, 1993). The need to preserve life at all costs continues to be the focus of medical science, this is where the psychosocial, spiritual and quality-of-life focus of palliative care clashes with conventional, acute medicine.

The traditional role of the nurse carrying out the doctor's orders has changed. With increasing knowledge and a research base, nursing as a profession is now more autonomous.

Whilst we still need to respect the position of the consultant in charge of the patient's care, we need to be able to give opinions based on our knowledge of the patient and family, and we need to involve ourselves in these decisions about the appropriateness of treatment. In the United States nurses have become very involved in the decision-making process and play a major role in the facilitation of choices about end of life care (American Nursing Association, 1991). The UK nursing organisations have not produced such detailed guidance as the American Nursing Association, but nurses should still be involved in such decision-making when appropriate to those in their care.

By becoming articulate, focusing on quality, rather than quantity of life, looking at the patient as a 'whole being', and taking account of their social and psychological well-being, the nurse will be in a better position to discuss treatment refusal.

Artificial nutrition and hydration

The provision of nutrition and hydration is a basic function of the nurse. As patients near death their interest in food and drink wanes and they often become too weak to feed themselves or to drink independently. In most cases the nurse will give assistance to those who are still able to eat and drink. However, problems can arise when the subject of artificial nutrition and hydration is raised. Artificial nutrition and hydration 'refers specifically to those techniques for providing nutrition or hydration which are used to bypass a pathology in the swallowing process. It includes the use of nasogastric tubes, percutaneous endoscopic gastrostomy (PEG feeding), and total parenteral nutrition' (BMA, 1999).

Many patients will already be receiving intravenous fluids as they approach the terminal stages of illness. The problem arises as to whether it is beneficial to carry on giving such fluids as patients continue through the terminal stages. Current thinking is that an assessment needs to be made of each individual's needs in relation to artificial hydration. One method of assessment that can be helpful is the one suggested by Zerwekh (1997):

- Is the patient's well-being enhanced by the overall effect of hydration?
- Which current symptoms are being relieved by artificial hydration?
- Are other end of life symptoms being aggravated by the fluids?
- Does hydration improve the patient's level of consciousness? If so, is this within the patient's goals and wishes for end of life care?
- Does it appear to prolong the patient's survival? If so, is this within the patient's goals and wishes for end of life care?
- What is the effect of the infusion technology on the patient's well-being, mobility, ability to interact and be with the family?
- What is the burden of the infusion technology on the family in terms of caregiver stress? Is it justified by benefit to the patient?

A number of studies have compared the need for hydration in the terminally ill. Bruera and Faisinger (1997) found that whilst some patients may benefit from dehydration, others with confusion or opioid toxicity might benefit from hydration. At St Christopher's Hospice a major study showed that there was no correlation between thirst and hydration (Ellershaw et al, 1995). Thirst is one of the main reasons given for continuing to give intravenous fluids! There is also the increased risk of fluid overload leading to pulmonary congestion and nausea and vomiting. Smith (1995) describes two studies that show longer survival times without hydration.

With all this in mind, we suggest that as with all end of life decisions, the patient, if able, the family and the multidisciplinary team should be involved in the decision to initiate or continue artificial hydration.

The concept of double effect

Medical care has a moral and ethical obligation to relieve pain and other distressing symptoms of advanced disease. Very often patients and carers will see the introduction of strong opiate drugs to control pain as the first step towards hastening death. This remains a common misconception amongst many cancer patients. It is of course the case that strong opiates have such an effect, but they are not used for this specific intent.

Palliative care aims to help the patient live as long as possible; when the patient's quality of life deteriorates and they reach a stage where death is imminent, it helps them to die, not too early or not too late. Those who must die are assured a death with dignity. As cancer advances the symptoms become more and more complex and distressing. The combination of drugs and other interventions very often includes increasing doses of opioid analgesics. There is a definite difference between giving drugs for the express purpose of relieving pain, and giving drugs to cause death. The recognition that strong opioids cause respiratory depression at higher doses, but are being used for their primary analgesic effect, is known as double effect.

It is important that those close to the patient are made aware that the primary aim of giving strong opioids is to relieve pain. Nurses should not avoid talking about double effect but it is vital that the family fully understand the concept in order to avoid concern and confusion.

Do not resuscitate orders

It is important that the subject of cardiopulmonary resuscitation (CPR) is discussed with cancer patients at a suitable stage of the illness. It is of course futile to consider CPR in anyone who is obviously in the terminal stages of their illness. In such cases there would be no hope of achieving a satisfactory outcome. Nurses should remember that one of the aims of palliative care is to allow the patient to die with dignity. CPR is not a very dignified procedure and it should not be necessary to document or discuss CPR in the patient who is obviously terminal.

However, patients might be admitted to an acute surgical or medical ward early in their illness. In such cases there needs to be a determined effort by the team to think about the possibility of sudden cardiorespiratory arrest, and what would be the best outcome for the patient. It is very often the nurse who will discover a collapsed patient and have to take the decision on whether or not to instigate CPR. It is neither fair nor appropriate to expect anyone to take such a decision at such a stressful time; therefore the decision needs to have been made as soon as possible after the patient's admission.

It is often a difficult choice of topic to raise with any patient, let alone those who know they have a life-threatening illness. Therefore, it is important that the time is right and that the medical staff are there to give support. It is also the ultimate responsibility of the consultant in charge of the case to verify the decision not to resuscitate. There needs to be a careful and full explanation of the possible outcomes of CPR, the effects on quality of life, and the real possibility of failure. The patient needs to be fully aware of this and is of course to be fully involved. Any objections by the patient or next of kin should preclude the DNR order being instituted, and an attempt at CPR must be made.

Euthanasia

Euthanasia is illegal in most Western countries. The law in the UK is quite clear – acts with the primary intention of causing the patient's death or the facilitation of suicide are forbidden. This is quite clear and unambiguous. Nurses will sometimes be faced with a patient who, despite palliative interventions, is in considerable distress. They may have intractable pain, or other distressing symptoms and are clearly suffering. In some cases the patient might beg to be 'put out of their misery', often making such pleas to the nurse. This is a particularly difficult situation to deal with and calls on the nurse's caring and communication skills. There is no place in these situations to even think about acting on the patient's wishes.

The nurse needs to be able to listen to the patient's fears and concerns. Unrelieved symptoms need to be dealt with by specialist input, and referral as appropriate. The patient might benefit from talking to a counsellor, minister of religion, or psychiatrist as the 'physical' symptoms often hide more deep-seated emotional or psychological hurt. The nurse who is dealing with a patient having such thoughts towards suicide or euthanasia also needs to consider their own support needs and should seek help from peers, or counselling, to ensure they cope and come through the experience.

CHAPTER 5

The Multi-professional Team

Palliative care by its very nature is a team effort. This chapter will give the reader insight into the roles of the different members of the team and how they can be best utilised to provide optimum care to cancer and palliative care patients.

Medical roles

Cancer patient come into contact with many different doctors during their illness. It might be their general practitioner, a hospital physician or surgeon or oncologist who initially breaks the news of their illness. Throughout their illness they will regularly come in contact with these specialists again. However, in palliative care their main contacts will be their general practitioner and the palliative care physician.

General practitioner (GP)

The general practitioner is a medical generalist and is generally considered to be the head of the primary care team.

He or she is usually responsible for approximately two thousand patients. The principal role of the GP is to prevent illness: diagnose disease and manage disease on a 24-hour basis. GPs are becoming increasingly involved in palliative care in the community and are responsible for those patients dying at home.

Palliative medicine specialist

These doctors have postgraduate training in the specialty of palliative care and are normally asked for advice regarding specific needs in palliative care. They are usually based in a hospice or specialist palliative care unit and are asked to see patients on a visiting basis.

They very often work as part of a hospital palliative care team in conjunction with clinical nurse specialists.

Nursing roles

Hospital nurses

Nurses working in acute settings such as medical, surgical or oncology wards are very much part of the multi-professional team. Their role in providing basic palliative care is vital. Acute nurses are very often the first to notice distressing symptoms and instigate appropriate interventions.

Specialist palliative care nurses

These nurses have usually gone on to complete specific post-registration training in oncology or palliative care. Many are termed Macmillan nurses in recognition of the Charity that pays for them. They usually work as part of a hospital palliative care team, but might also be hospice based.

Macmillan nurses are advisers and do not get involved in 'hands on' nursing. Within the hospital they will assess patients' palliative care needs and give advice on symptom control, nursing management etc., in conjunction with the palliative care consultant.

District nurses

The district nurse's role in palliative care is expanding owing to improved supportive care for cancer patients. Many people are living longer with the disease and want to be at home either for extensive periods, or in many cases to die. This means that their care needs are ever more complex and that planning for home care takes time and effort. This is something that hospital nurses need to take heed of when discharging such patients.

Other health care professionals

Physiotherapists

The usual role of the physiotherapists involves them in restoring normal musculoskeletal function, prevention of deformity and the prevention of complications such as chest infection postoperatively. Within cancer and palliative care they have additional roles. They aim to maximise and maintain the patient's decreasing physical resources. They are often involved in symptom control, e.g. lymphoedema management, chest drainage and neuropathic pain management, using TENS (transcutaneous electrical nerve stimulation) machines, exercises etc. They can provide education and aids to maintaining mobility and are excellent resource for both nurses and carers, giving advice on moving and handling. Many are involved with therapeutic massage, which not only relaxes and improves blood flow, but also is an excellent opportunity to talk and listen to people. Specialist palliative care physiotherapy is a growing interest.

Occupational therapists

Occupational therapists (OTs) often work closely with physiotherapists. Their main role is in maximising patients' safe, independent living potential. OTs perform detailed assessments of the person's ability to carry out daily living tasks such as feeding, dressing and mobilising. They provide adaptations and aids to enhance and maintain these skills. They are an excellent source of help to patients, carers and staff. They have close connections with community services and will often visit patients' homes to assess needs and provide the necessary adaptations to bathing and dressing etc.

The OT's traditional role is seen by many nurses as organising bingo, macramé or basket weaving. This role is now carried out by diversional therapists, mainly based in hospices and trained outside the health service.

Dieticians

Adequate nutrition is essential when someone has cancer. Not only does the treatment have an effect on nutritional status, e.g. chemotherapy induced nausea, but also the disease itself causes an increase in the body's nutritional requirements.

The dietician's specialist knowledge and experience allows them to make a detailed assessment of patients' individual needs and how the best to advise them. They can provide not only individual meal choices but also supplements and to the patients' taste.

Dieticians are involved in the later stages of illness when the quality of life issues become more of a focus than nutrition as such. They also work closely with speech therapists and language therapists to manage swallowing problems; if these occur then nasogastric feeding/parenteral feeding are also options.

Pharmacists

The clinical pharmacist's role extends far beyond the provision of medicines. They are a valuable source of information to patients, families and carers. Their detailed knowledge of pharmacology means they can advise on possible side effects or drug interactions and best combinations to avoid these. When drugs are being administered via subcutaneous syringe driver and combinations are being given, the pharmacist's advice is usually invaluable.

Increasingly pharmacists involved in cancer and palliative care are given further specialist training and knowledge.

Social workers

The social worker's role is to help the patient, family and carers to deal effectively with the personal and social problems of cancer and impending death.

Social workers are employed by the local council and work in both the hospital and community. They can provide patients and their family with advice on financial matters and benefits. Special benefits allow patients with terminal illness prompt access to attendance allowance and disability living allowance. The social worker will also assess the need for community care support such as meals on wheels, home help, bathing etc. They work closely with occupational therapists in decisions about any necessary adaptations, as it is usually the local council who carry out these changes. Social workers are also closely involved with counselling and bereavement support for families.

Chaplains

Chaplains are excellent talkers but are also trained to listen. They can be an excellent resource to help both patients and carers. As we saw in Chapter 3, many patients experience a huge range of emotions and many people turn to religion during this period.

Many patients when they feel that the terminal stage is approaching will have a need to know what lies ahead of them. Some will fear what is to come and need help to come to terms with it. This is a time when the chaplain's help is invaluable. Once the patient has died the chaplain can usually be relied on to comfort and care for the bereaved family.

CHAPTER 6

Communication in Cancer and Palliative Care

Communication is a basic need in any health care setting, and is particularly important in cancer and palliative care. Unfortunately, it is still not as good as it should be. In this chapter the authors look at the issues of basic listening skills – what we do wrong, and what we should be doing when listening to patients and carers. How do we as nurses manage communication within the multi-professional team? And how do we go about breaking bad news?

Listening to patients and carers

Stedeford (1981) states that poor communication is a bigger problem to cancer patients and their families than physical symptoms, with the exemption of pain. Any communication involves the transmission or sharing of a message or information between a sender and a receiver. Very often cancer patients have complex communication issues and active listening is vital if we are to respond effectively to these needs. Active listening helps to support not only the patient but also the family, who are just as much our responsibility as the patient. Active listening will also cut down on wasted time and helps to build better relationships (Straka, 1997). Active listening also involves being able to interpret and respond to the individual's body language and non-verbal communication. This becomes easier with experience and as the relationship with the patient and family strengthens.

Active listening is very helpful at removing barriers to effective care. One of the main ones is a fear of pain and the use of morphine. Many patients will see the use of morphine as a last resort and will express fears about it hastening death. Listening carefully to such fears and trying to find out what lies behind them is important; it is not simply a matter of telling the patient that this is not the case. It is common for cancer patients to be given information booklets, and there are many hundreds available. Once patients have had time to read through them, nurses need to employ their own knowledge and skills to answer any questions patients may have in relation to the information they have read, or been given. Active listening on the nurse's part is vital at this stage.

Active listening also involves the use of open ended questions, which allow the patient to elaborate on what they are saying, rather than closed questions, which allow only 'yes/no' answers. This is a skill that comes with experience and time, and once again becomes easier as the therapeutic relationship develops.

Multi-professional team communication

Earlier we saw how palliative care involves multi-professional teamwork. This very often can lead to poor communication with such a diverse number of specialists looking after the patient and family. Very often the medical consultant is seen as head of the 'team' and this can in some cases be the cause of poor communication. How many of us remember the ward round where the consultant, registrar, senior house officer, house officer, ward sister and staff nurse march around from one bed to the next? The patient gets a cursory 'Good morning Mr Smith', a quick examination and a 'Good show!' and then the entourage moves on to the next patient. This is no longer an acceptable method of communicating, especially where cancer patients are concerned.

There needs to be meaningful communication between the whole team, and this is probably best achieved by holding regular team meetings to discuss the patients under the care of the team. It is normal for such meetings to feature the whole team and they are an excellent forum for ensuring that the patient and family are receiving optimum care. This type of meeting also means that the appropriate specialist can become involved as and when needed. The patient and family then only see a limited number of people and this can cut down on the feeling that the patient is losing control, which is a common feeling in cancer patients. Close communication also means that accurate needs assessments are made and this again cuts down on unnecessary intervention.

Breaking bad news

Increasingly within palliative care nurses are becoming involved in breaking bad news to patients and their families. This can be a difficult time not only for the person getting the bad news, but also for the person breaking it. Buckman (1998) suggests the following six-step protocol for breaking bad news, which readers might find helpful:

1. Getting the physical context right.
2. Finding out how much the patient knows.
3. Finding out how much the patient wants to know.
4. Sharing information (aligning and educating).
5. Responding to the patient's feelings.
6. Planning and following through.

Getting the physical context right

This means planning ahead to decide the best place to tell the patient. The middle of a busy ward with the screens pulled around the bed is not the most appropriate place to tell anyone any news never mind bad news. It is best to take the patient and family member to a comfortable, private room. The seating needs to be informal, usually with the patient and family member side by side facing the person breaking the news. Its also a good idea to have some tissues to hand. It is important *never* to break bad news to anyone sitting behind a desk, as this puts up a barrier between you and the patient that will be difficult to break down.

Finding out how much the patient knows

Again, open questioning is the best way to find out what patients already know about their illness. Questions such as 'Have you been worried about yourself lately?', 'What sort of symptoms have you had?', 'What did you think might be causing them?' will help you to find out a great deal about what the patients already know or suspect about their illness. It is very important for you to know what a patient thinks before you start to talk about the present and future, as it will have a bearing on what you eventually say.

Finding out how much the patient wants to know

Some patients may tell you what they know, and then say that is all they want to know. It is important at this stage to follow these wishes and comply, as this might be how the patient is coping with the illness at this time. Also remember that the patient is your main focus of attention. In some cases the patient does not wish to know, but the family are desperate to know. You should ensure that you are given the patient's permission to tell the family, and never tell them anything that the patient does not want them to know.

Sharing information (aligning and educating)

This is a two-part process for imparting medical information. Aligning is the reinforcement stage after finding out what the patient knows. After actively listening to the patient, the person breaking the bad news reinforces the positive aspects of the conversation. This gives the patient some confidence that what he said is correct and helps move the conversation forward.

Educating involves taking the conversation forward by providing the detailed medical information that patients need to have a better understanding of the future. It is at this point that patients should be told about their detailed diagnosis, treatment plans and possible outcomes. It is unhelpful to talk about prognosis at this point and it is rarely something that oncologists will discuss.

Responding to the patient's feelings

In most cases the patient will usually respond in a similar way – many will be relieved that the feelings they had have been confirmed, and that they can now go forward. Others will react with tears, either shocked or relieved. The patient's reaction will dictate how you should respond. Some people will react with another barrage of questions, some will go silent and say nothing. Whatever reaction the patient has, you need to be able to respond. This is something that comes with experience.

Planning and following through

Once you have responded appropriately to the patient, the interview needs to be closed. This is best achieved by agreeing with the patient what has been discussed. What is going to happen next, i.e. investigations, treatment, palliative care etc.? What information or further needs does the patient or family have? It is also helpful to provide the patient or family member with a contact point either for yourself if appropriate or for the ward/unit, so that should they have any further questions or information needs, they can get in touch.

Chapter 7
The Management of Cancer Pain

When thinking about the symptoms of cancer most if not all of us will think of pain first.

Bonica (1987) reports that 30–40% of patients will have pain at diagnosis, 30–40% at the intermediate stage of the disease and 60–100% depending on the site of the tumour at the advanced stage of disease.

The International Association for the Study of Pain (IASP, 1986) defined pain thus: 'Pain is an unpleasant sensory and emotional experience associated with actual or potential tissue damage.'

This is followed by a note stating that pain is a subjective, individual experience and that we must also take into account the psychological dimension of pain.

McCaffrey and Beebe (1994) also talk about the body's total response to pain, as illustrated in Figure 7.1.

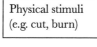

```
┌─────────────────────┐
│ Physical stimuli    │
│ (e.g. cut, burn)    │
└─────────────────────┘                        ┌──────────────────────────────┐
                                                │ Pain                         │
         +                    =                 │ (pain perception/intensity   │
                                                │ or pain tolerance)           │
┌─────────────────────┐                        └──────────────────────────────┘
│ Mental stimuli      │
│ (e.g. emotion, thought) │
└─────────────────────┘
```

Figure 7.1. The body's total response to pain.

Pain types

Cervero (1991) describes three types of pain.

1. Physiological.
2. Pathological.
3. Neuropathic.

Physiological pain

This is seen as a warning of potential tissue damage, e.g. pain in the muscles of the lower back when we sit at an awkward angle. The pain is usually sudden and in relation to the potential or actual tissue damage; e.g. when we drink something that is too hot the pain usually lasts for a few seconds.

Pathological pain

This is probably the most frequent type of pain experienced by cancer patients. Pathological pain is caused by a persistent painful stimulus or actual tissue damage. It is usually caused by tumour growth and spread, the release of noxious chemicals or chronic inflammation. Pathological pain is also known as chronic pain.

Neuropathic pain

This type of pain results from nerve damage and leads to alterations in normal pain perception. The pain can be as a result of the tumour pressing against or infiltrating a nerve, or as a side effect of treatment – radiotherapy, chemotherapy, surgery. A clear indication of neuropathic pain is when a seemingly innocuous stimulus such as a light, cold or heat leads to extreme pain (allodynia).

Neuropathic pain is the most difficult to treat.

The concept of total pain

The first stage in the management of cancer pain is accurate assessment of the causes of the pain. In cancer patients this can be difficult as there are so many probable causes. Effective assessment and use of analgesia can treat 80% of cancer pain simply and easily. Figure 7.2 shows the factors that contribute to the patient's total pain.

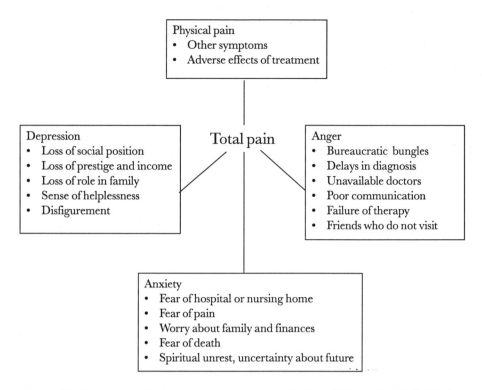

Figure 7.2. Factors contributing to the patient's total pain. From Fallan and O'Neill (1998).

The World Health Organization (WHO) three-step ladder

Analgesic drugs are the mainstay of cancer pain management. The choice drug should relate to the severity of pain and should be based on the three-step ladder proposed by the WHO (1996) (Figure 7.3).

The principle is that for mild pain a non-opioid should be used, building up to an opioid and adjuvant for severe pain. The drugs commonly recommended for cancer pain are:

Mild pain:

- Aspirin 600 mg every 4 hours.
- Paracetamol 1 g every 4 hours.

Moderate pain:

- Codeine 60 mg (+ non-opioid) every 4 hours.
- Dextropropoxyphene 65 mg (+ non-opioid) every 4 hours.

Severe pain:

• Morphine 5–10 mg (starting dose) every 4 hours.

Ideally these drugs should be given by mouth every 4 hours without fail. Only breakthrough pain occurring within the 4 hours should be treated on a 'PRN' (as required) basis.

An adjuvant is a drug whose primary effect is not pain relief but has analgesic effect in some conditions, e.g. non-steroidal anti-inflammatory drugs, tricyclic antidepressants, anticonvulsants. The aim of the WHO ladder is broad spectrum analgesia and drugs from each the three classes of analgesic mentioned, i.e. non-opioid, opioid, adjuvant, should be used, either singly or in combination to achieve the desired effect. However, care needs to be taken to avoid patients being prescribed multiple drugs with no positive effects.

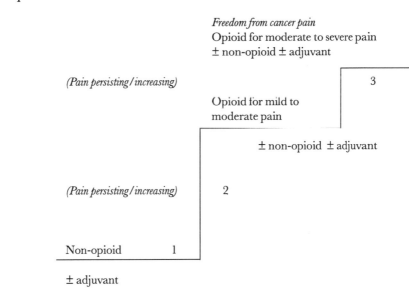

Freedom from cancer pain
Opioid for moderate to severe pain
± non-opioid ± adjuvant

(Pain persisting/increasing)   3

Opioid for mild to
moderate pain

± non-opioid ± adjuvant

(Pain persisting/increasing)   2

Pain   Non-opioid   1

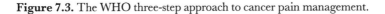

± adjuvant

Figure 7.3. The WHO three-step approach to cancer pain management.

Non-opioids

Paracetamol

Paracetamol is indicated in mild to moderate pain and in pyrexia (antipyretic). It is a synthetic non-opioid analgesic which inhibits prostaglandin synthesis. The antipyretic action is a result of the inhibition of the hypothalamic heat regulatory centre.

Paracetamol is well tolerated, even in peptic ulceration. Adverse side effects within normal dose limits are rare and it does not injure gastric mucosa.

The normal dose in adults is 1 g every 4 – 6 hours; maximum dose is 4 g in 24 hours (orally). By rectum the dose is 1 g up to four times daily.

Presentation:

500 mg tablets
120 mg/5 ml elixir
125 mg suppositories.

Side effects mainly relate to drug overdose and include nausea, vomiting, abdominal pain; progressive liver toxicity leads to death.

Care should be taken in patients with liver disease, kidney disease and chronic alcohol problems.

Non-steroidal anti-inflammatory drugs (NSAIDs)

NSAIDS are particularly useful in pathological pain caused by actual tissue damage, e.g. tumour infiltration and bone metastases. They can also play a part in controlling neuropathic pain (Ripamonti et al, 1996). The most commonly used drugs in palliative care are naproxen, diclofenac and ibruprofen.

Diclofenac

Diclofenac is indicated in mild to moderate pain particularly associated with tissue inflammation.

It inhibits prostaglandin synthesis and is anti-inflammatory; like most NSAIDs it is not well tolerated in patients with peptic ulceration and those allergic to aspirin. It can cause damage to gastric mucosa.

The normal dose is 25–50 mg every 8–12 hours; modified release (MR) tablets are available as 100 mg daily or 75 mg once or twice daily. Rectally, the dose is 75–150 mg, usually at night.

Presentation:

25 mg and 50 mg enteric coated tablets
75 mg and 100 mg MR tablets
50 mg dispersible tablets
12.5 mg and 100 mg suppositories
75 mg/3 ml intramuscular injection.

Side effects include nausea, anorexia, vomiting, diarrhoea, jaundice, peptic ulceration and gastrointestinal bleeding, dizziness fatigue, nephrotoxicity and haematuria. Care needs to be taken in patients sensitive to aspirin, or with active peptic ulceration or gastric ulceration bleeding.

Naproxen

Naproxen is indicated in the mild to moderate pain particularly associated with tissue inflammation.

It inhibits prostaglandin synthesis by decreasing an enzyme needed for biosynthesis and is anti-inflammatory.

It is not well tolerated by people with peptic ulcer, asthma or sensitivity to aspirin.

Normal dose is 25–500 mg twice daily or 500 mg rectally at night.

Presentation:

250 mg and 500 mg tablets
500 mg MR tablets
125 mg/5 ml suspension
500 mg suppositories

Side effects are as for Diclofenac.

Ibuprofen

Ibuprofen is indicated in mild to moderate pain particularly associated with tissue inflammation.

It inhibits prostaglandin synthesis by decreasing an enzyme needed for biosynthesis and is anti-inflammatory. It is not well tolerated by people with peptic ulcer, asthma or sensitivity to aspirin.

Normal dose is 1.2–1.8 g daily in three to four doses; not available as a suppository.

Presentation:

200 mg and 400 mg tablets
800 mg MR tablets
100 mg/5 ml syrup
600 mg/sachet effervescent granules.

Side effects are as for diclofenac.

The NSAIDs also have an antipyretic action and can reduce neoplastic fever, but at the present time they are not licensed for such use in the United Kingdom.

Weak opioids

Weak opioids given by intramuscular (IM) injection can provide analgesia equivalent or healing equivalent to 10 mg morphine (Twycross, Wilcock and Thorp, 1998).

Codeine phosphate

Codeine phosphate is a weak opioid analgesic which acts on the central nervous system opiate receptors and inhibits the ascending pain pathways. It reduces gastrointestinal motility.

It is indicated in pain unrelieved by non-opioids, diarrhoea and cough.

Normal dose for analgesia is 30–60 mg every 4 hours by mouth, up to a daily maximum of 240 mg, or 30–60 mg every 4 hours by IM injection.

Presentation:

60 mg/ml injection
15, 30, 60 mg tablets
15 mg/5 ml and 25 mg/5 ml syrup.

Side effects include drowsiness, sedation, dizziness, agitation, nausea, vomiting, constipation. In the elderly lung it may also cause cardiac arrhythmias and increased intracranial pressure.

Dextropropoxyphene (co-proxamol)

A weak opioid analgesic, dextropropoxyphene is a synthetic derivative of methadone. It is similar in action to codeine.

It is indicated in moderate to severe pain unrelieved by non-opioids alone.

Normal dose is two tablets (as Co-proxamol) every 4 hours or as required; maximum of eight tables per day as this is a compound that contains paracetamol (UK).

Presentation:

Co-proxamol 32.5/325 tablets (32.5 mg dextropropoxyphene hydrochloride/325 mg paracetamol)
65 mg dextropropoxyphene hydrochloride capsules.

Side effects are as for codeine plus it may enhance the effects of oral anti-coagulants, carbamazepine and alcohol.

Dihydrocodeine (DF118)

Dihydrocodeine, a synthetic derivative of codeine, is a weak opioid.
It is indicated in moderate to severe pain, cough and diarrhoea.
Normal dose in pain control is 30 mg every 4–6 hours.
Presentation:

30 mg tablets
60 mg MR tablets
10 mg/5 ml syrup
50 mg/ml injection (Controlled Drug).

Side effects are as for codeine.

Strong opioids

Morphine

Morphine is the strong opioid of choice throughout the world (WHO, 1996). Strong opioids inhibit the ascending pain pathways in the central nervous system, increase the pain threshold and alter pain perception.

They are indicated in severe pain, both acute and chronic.

In the management of cancer pain morphine should be given in conjunction with a non-opioid (Twycross et al, 1998).

Normal dose is 5–20 mg every 4 hours. Modified release tablets are normally given in cancer patients. The previous daily dose of morphine is noted and then divided by two and given every 12 hours.

By rectum the dose is 15–30 mg every 4 hours.
Presentation:

10, 15, 30 mg injection
10 mg/5 ml; 100 mg/5 ml oral solution
10 mg/5 ml; 30 mg/5 ml; 100 mg/5 ml unit dose vials
5, 10, 15, 30, 60, 100 mg sachets
5, 10, 20, 30, 60, 100, 200 mg morphine sustained release (MST).

For side effects see Table 7.1.

Diamorphine

Diamorphine is a strong opioid analgesic generally used in severe pain, particularly in terminal care. It is usually used instead of morphine parenterally in the UK.

Normal dose is 5–10 mg every 4 hours, increased according to need. IM dose should be approximately half the oral dose for the same level of pain.
Presentation:

10 mg tablets
5, 10, 30, 100 and 500 mg powder for injection.

For side effects see Table 7.1.

Table 7.1. Side effects of strong opioids (Twycross et al, 1998)

Common initial
Nausea and vomiting
Drowsiness
Unsteadiness
Delirium (confusion)

Common ongoing
Constipation
Nausea and vomiting

Occasional
Dry mouth
Sweating
Pruritus
Hallucinations

Rare
Respiratory depression
Psychological dependence

Management of pain without drugs

Whilst drugs remain the first line approach to the management of acute pain, many other non-pharmacological approaches have been used in the management of chronic pain in association with drugs. The main areas we will look at in this chapter are:

- massage;
- heat and cold application;
- TENS;
- aromatherapy.

Massage

Massage can be defined as 'stimulation of the skin and underlying tissues with varying degrees of hand pressure to decrease pain, produce relaxation and/or improve circulation' (Mobily et al, 1994).

Massage has been used as a therapy for many thousands of years.

As well as the feeling of warmth and comfort due to increases in capillary circulation, muscle relaxation and distraction, the interaction between the patient and operator through touch has immeasurable benefits.

The most common areas of the body to be massaged are the hands, face and neck, the back or shoulders. Whilst nurses can be trained and authorised to carry out certain types of massage, e.g. hands or feet, it is usual for a physiotherapist to carry out massage as a therapy. In long-term cancer patients it is sometimes possible to teach the family to carry out hand/feet massage. There have been some concerns expressed about the possibility of massage 'spreading' cancer around the body (McNamarra, 1994). However, there is no evidence to support this belief (Hawthorn and Redmond, 1999). It is not advisable to massage over a palpable tumour or radiotherapy treatment sites.

As with many effective complementary therapies, there is little scientific evidence to support its use in the management of cancer pain. Sims (1986) and Ferrel-Torry and Glick (1993) carried out small-scale studies of massage in cancer patients and found decreases in pain reported by the patients involved. This is enough evidence for the nurse to consider the use of massage as an adjuvant therapy in pain management.

Heat and cold application

The application of heat and cold has also been used for centuries. It is a simple and effective intervention for pain. Radiant heat applied by a lamp, immersion in water or by pads of various kinds causes an increase in blood flow which increases oxygenation. It is thought that the increased blood flow also removes pain-carrying substances.

Heat is very helpful when dealing with musculoskeletal problems, such as spasms, joint stiffness, back pain, and with menstrual problems. As with massage, the physiotherapist is the main person to contact about the use of heat and cold. Nurses must be sure to prevent injury from the heating device and need to supervise patients closely if physiotherapist has devolved responsibility for treatment.

The application of cold reduces swelling and the amount of metabolites in tissues by vasoconstriction (Ernst and Fialka, 1994). Cold is thought to be more effective than heat and can reduce muscle spasms and joint stiffness. Cold can be applied via icepacks, immersion in cold water or ice ethylchloride spray or a cold compress.

Heat and cold can be used interchangeably and this is probably the best way to manage pain.

TENS (transcutaneous electrical nerve stimulation)

TENS is a method of pain control which uses low voltage electrical current from electrodes placed on the skin. TENS consists of a small control box, wires and skin electrodes. The electrodes are placed over the site of the pain (skin must be intact) and connected to the control box via the leads. The electrodes must be coated in the conducting jelly first. Once in place and switched on, the patient experiences sensations of vibration, tingling or pulsating. The patient is told how to reposition the electrodes for maximum effect.

The strength, pattern, period and rate of the impulses can be changed for the best results (Davis, 2000).

TENS is particularly effective in chronic pain, including neurogenic pain (Bates and Nathan, 1980). It is usually administered by physiotherapists or specially trained nurses. TENS should not be used if the patient has a pacemaker, or on the neck or in pregnancy.

Aromatherapy

Aromatherapy uses essential plant oils for their therapeutic effects (Stevenson, 1995). These oils are applied by massage in a plain carrier oil such as grape-seed oil. The oils can also be used as vapours, bath water or as compress. Many nurses are now doing further training in the use of aromatherapy, even though the scientific evidence is limited. It is important to note that aromatherapy is contraindicated in children and the very ill adult (McNamarra, 1994).

The following essential oils have analgesic, antispasmodic and anti-inflammatory properties:

- lavender;
- Roman camomile;
- rosemary;
- ginger;
- myrrh;
- bergamot.

It is vital that appropriate training has been completed before using aromatherapy in analgesia.

Radiotherapy in the management of pain

Radiotherapy is a useful tool in the management of pain caused by metastases. It can be administered either by teletherapy (external beam) or as a radioisotope. The most common tumours to spread to bone are breast, bronchus or prostate. Headache resulting from brain metastases may also respond to radiotherapy.

External beam radiotherapy

Radiotherapy is a very effective treatment for pain caused by bone metastases. Worthwhile pain relief is achieved in about 65% of patients and 20% have complete pain relief (Yarnold, 1995).

Patients with bone metastases usually undergo what is called hemibody irradiation. The patient is admitted to a radiotherapy unit usually the day before treatment. The patient is usually given a large dose of radiation which kills metastatic cells and so relieves pain. This is opposite to the usual carefully directed beam which is used normally in cancer management. Such a large dose of radiation can lead to severe nausea and vomiting; therefore patients are given intravenous (IV) fluids and IV anti-emetics prior to treatment.

Brain metastases usually cause pain (headache) the same as any other space-occupying lesion. Radiotherapy is usually given as a wide field or total brain irradiation at a small dose. This treatment is usually palliative, i.e. not aimed at cure, but many patients go on to survive many months.

Radioisotopes

Radioisotopes such as strontium (^{89}Sr) relieve pain by concentrating in areas of osteoblast activity. The dose and therefore area of action is based within the area of uptake.

Strontium can be given on an out-patient basis or the patient is admitted overnight for observation. The isotope is given by injection (IV) and there are usually no side effects. The radiation is concentrated in the site of the bone metastases, so the patient is not a radiation risk, unlike patients given iodine-131.

Patients with long-term bone pain may have both strontium and hemi-body irradiation over a period of time.

Syringe drivers in pain management

A syringe driver is a battery-operated device that moves the plunger of a syringe at a controlled rate. It is usually used to deliver drugs over a 24-hour period. The most commonly used syringe drivers are the Graseby MS16A and MS26 models. Both of these models are portable and can be used to deliver drugs by the subcutaneous or intravenous routes.

The syringe driver is used when the oral route is inappropriate or the patient is unable to swallow due to:

- intestinal obstruction;
- nausea and/or vomiting;
- malabsorption;
- mouth, throat or oesophageal lesions;
- weakness/unconsciousness;
- terminal stage of illness.

The syringe driver can be used to deliver the following analgesics by the subcutaneous route: diamorphine, fentanyl, morphine.

Continuous infusion has a number of benefits over IM injections, such as a reduction in plasma concentration variations, avoidance of injections, and the patient can still be mobile as long as required.

The syringe driver can be used to deliver mixtures of drugs to control symptoms and these are described in more detail in Chapter 11.

Detailed instructions on the use of syringe drivers can be obtained from: Sims Graseby Limited, Colonial Way, Watford WD2 4LG, UK.

CHAPTER 8

Managing Distressing Symptoms

As cancer progresses and treatment becomes more aggressive, the distressing side effects and symptoms tend to increase. In this chapter the authors have identified some of the more common side effects and symptoms that might be seen in patients with advanced cancer. The pathophysiology, nursing assessment, nursing and medical management will be described. The symptoms covered are:

- nausea and vomiting;
- dysphagia;
- bowel obstruction;
- diarrhoea and constipation;
- mouth problems;
- lymphoedema;
- dyspnoea;
- ascites and pleural effusion.

Nausea and vomiting

Nausea is a subjective experience associated with many different causes. It is normally associated with retching and precedes vomiting. Vomiting is the forced emptying of the stomach through the mouth. Projective vomiting is vomiting not preceded by nausea or retching and is an indication of stimulation of the vomiting centre in the brain usually by a tumour or increased intracranial pressure.

Nausea and vomiting are common in cancer patients. Studies (Baines, 1988; Lindley and Hirsch, 1992; Martin, 1992) have shown that 50% of patients experience nausea and vomiting as a consequence of cancer treatment, whilst disease processes of cancer, e.g. bowel obstruction, are responsible for the other 50%.

Treatment-induced nausea and vomiting

Most chemotherapy agents can be implicated in inducing nausea. This is most common in the early stages of drug administration and infusion. However, drugs such as cisplatin (platinum) can produce nausea and vomiting that lasts several days.

Barnes and Barnes (1991) identified the pathways implicated in cytotoxic related nausea and vomiting.

The area postrema is found in the brainstem and is the location for the chemoreceptor trigger zone. It lies outwith the blood–brain barrier and is part of the systemic circulation. Dopamine receptors are stimulated by high concentrations of emetogenic substances (Twycross, 1997).

The main connection of the vagus nerve lies in the area postrema. The emetic pattern generator is inside the blood–brain barrier and in the deep layers of the area postrema. As well as being stimulated by chemotherapy agents, the area postrema is affected by opioids.

Cancer-induced nausea and vomiting

Nausea and vomiting as a result of the disease itself, e.g. stomach cancer, intestinal obstruction, constipation, is more difficult to manage. It may involve the use of surgery or radiotherapy as well as drug management.

Nursing assessment of nausea and vomiting

An understanding of the cause of nausea and vomiting is the first step in the process of assessment. The pattern of nausea and vomiting can give valuable information on the cause post-chemotherapy, after eating. Accurate fluid balance and details about volume, content and nature of vomit can also give an indication as to the cause of vomiting. Biochemical analysis is usually undertaken and the doctor will carry out a detailed clinical examination.

Patients need to be asked about specific causes of nausea and vomiting, e.g. specific smells, tastes, sights, as these can be important factors in treatment or prevention of nausea and vomiting.

Management of nausea and vomiting

The mainstay of management of nausea and vomiting is drug treatment. The choice of drug depends on the cause of nausea and vomiting.

Prokinetic drugs

These enhance the tissue response to acetylcholine which causes contraction of the stomach muscle, relaxation of the pylorus and duodenal segment and increasing peristalsis. They also act on the chemoreceptor trigger zone by inhibiting dopamine receptors.

These drugs include:

Metoclopramide 30–80 mg (in 24 hours)
Domperidone 30–80 mg (in 24 hours)
Cisapride 20–30 mg (in 24 hours),

Antihistamines

Antihistamines such as cyclizine (150 mg/24 hours) act on the vestibular and vomiting centres in the brain and are particularly useful in radiation-induced nausea and vomiting.

Phenothiazines

Phenothiazines block dopamine at the chemoreceptor trigger zone, depress the cerebral cortex and act on the vestibular and vomiting centres. All of these actions lead to weakness and drowsiness, side effects that are useful in terminal care (see Chapter 11) but can be unhelpful in daily use. Methotrimeprazine (Nozinan) is the usual drug of choice and the daily dose is 12.5–75 mg.

Butyrophenones

Butyrophenones are drugs that depress the cerebral cortex and inhibit dopamine at the synapse. The action and side effects are similar to the phenothiazines. The commonest drug is haloperidol 1–2 mg per day.

$5HT_3$ receptor antagonists

These drugs act by antagonising the action of serotonin at receptors in the central nervous system, thereby intervening in the role serotonin plays in stimulating nausea and vomiting. Ondansetron (Zofran) is widely used as prophylaxis in chemotherapy- and radiotherapy-induced nausea and vomiting. The normal dose is 8 mg every 12 hours. Granisetron (Kytril) is the other common drug of this group used in chemotherapy and is given as a 3 mg infusion up to a maximum of 9 mg per day.

Corticosteroids

Corticosteroids such as dexamethasone reduce oedema and have a central and peripheral anti-emetic effect. They are particularly useful in chemotherapy-induced nausea and vomiting, where the usual regimen is 5–20 mg IV, 30 minutes before chemotherapy and 2–4 mg three times a day orally.

Anticholinergics

Anticholinergics act by inhibiting acetylcholine, which reduces gastrointestinal secretions and motility. The most common drug in oncology is hyoscine butylbromide 60–200 mg per day.

Non-drug management

Whilst drugs remain the mainstay of management there are other things that nurses can do to manage nausea and vomiting. These include simple measures such as helping the patient to avoid sights and smells that are unpleasant and could lead to nausea and vomiting. Small frequent meals that the patient likes should be encouraged in order to maintain nutritional needs. This is a situation where it is appropriate to involve the dietician in the management of the patient's symptoms.

Other non-pharmacological interventions that can be considered include relaxation techniques and distractions. There are already many audiotapes/CDs available which include relaxing music, nature sounds and spoken voice. These can be given to the patient along with a personal cassette/CD player, which the individual can use. Some people find this very helpful.

Acupressure using proprietary wrist bands with a button placed over the p6 point of the dominant arm has been shown to be effective in some cases. Wickham (1999) found that such wrist bands used in conjunction with the drug ondansetron were more effective than ondansetron alone.

Nausea and vomiting is a problem in cancer patients. However, with careful assessment and treatment it can be relieved.

Dysphagia

Dysphagia is difficulty in swallowing and is common in patients with cancer of the head and neck, oesophagus and stomach. Table 8.1 shows the three stages of swallowing and the causes of dysphagia in each of these stages.

The first stage of swallowing takes place in the mouth and is called the buccal phase. Once chewed and moistened the food bolus is pushed backward into the pharynx by the tongue and palate. The main causes of dysphagia at this stage are tumours of the tongue, uvula or palate, infection with *Candida albicans* (thrush), stomatitis caused by chemotherapy or radiotherapy and nervous dysfunction as a consequence of previous surgery or brainstem involvement.

The next stage occurs in the pharynx where the swallowing reflex initiates closure of the glottis. Once again, the main causes of dysphagia at this stage are tumours of the pharynx, vocal cords or larynx and glottic lesions. There can also be compression from tumours outside the pharynx, e.g. bronchial lesions or neck node swelling. Infection, radiotherapy and nerve damage are also implicated.

The final stage is the oesophageal phase, where food is passed down the oesophagus by peristalsis. Tumours, either intraluminal or extraluminal, are the main cause of dysphagia at this stage. Infection and radiotherapy and chemotherapy are the major factors.

Table 8.1. The causes of dysphagia at different levels of swallowing

Phase of swallowing	Causes of dysphagia
Buccal (mouth) phase	Tumour, candida, mucositis, radiotherapy, chemotherapy
Pharyngeal (throat) phase	Tumour, infection, radiotherapy
Oesophageal phase	Tumour (either in or outside lumen), infection, surgery, reflux

Nursing assessment of dysphagia

The first step in assessing dysphagia is to examine the patient's mouth. Special attention needs to be given to the general appearance of the gums and teeth – are there any signs of bleeding? The nature and the amount of saliva present – is it normal, thick or absent? Is the mouth dry and sore (mucositis)? Any signs of infection need to be noted: white spots/plaque indicate candida infection. Obvious lesions need to be noted and recorded.

Giving the patient sips of water and watching how they swallow can assess swallowing. Any problems such as coughing, regurgitation or aspiration need to be referred to a speech therapist. Obviously patients with dysphagia are at risk of nutritional deficits. Patients need to be referred to the dietician for a full nutritional assessment. Nurses must maintain accurate food records as well as documenting the state of the mouth.

Management of dysphagia

As with most management plans the treatment of dysphagia is dependent on the underlying cause.

Tumours

Tumours causing dysphagia either by direct mechanical obstruction or by pressure/invasion need to be treated in the usual way, i.e. surgery, chemotherapy, radiotherapy. Dexamethasone 8–12 mg orally can help reduce swelling and sometimes relieve dysphagia. Oesophageal dilation and stenting are common procedures used to relieve tumour obstruction in the oesophagus.

Candidiasis

This is an opportunistic infection usually seen in the mouth, but it can extend down the oesophagus in extreme cases. It is caused by yeast, usually *Candida albicans*, and is common in cancer patients.

The main causes of candida infection are corticosteroids, drugs and radiotherapy. The main clinical features are white plagues on a red swollen base (tongue, gums, mouth). Patients often complain of a dry metallic taste in the mouth. Removal of the plaques leads to bleeding, leaving the surface raw and sore.

Treatment involves careful and regular oral hygiene, denture cleaning and disinfection, and brushing. Antifungal agents such as fluconazole 50 mg daily for 7–14 days or ketoconazole 200 mg daily for 14 days may be prescribed. Chlorhexidine mouthwash is usually prescribed, as it has anti-fungal, antibacterial and slight antiviral properties. Extensive candida involving the oesophagus is usually treated with intravenous fluconazole.

Radiation mucositis

The mucous membranes are rapidly reproducing and are therefore particularly susceptible to damage from radiotherapy. The mucous membranes of the mouth become red and swollen and painful. Management includes careful oral hygiene with saline mouthwashes, sodium bicarbonate solution rinses and chlorhexidine mouthwash. The pain associated with mucositis is usually treated with drugs such as Mucaine, which is a combination of antacid and topical local anaesthetic.

Patients should be given advice on avoiding hot or cold foods or drinks; spicy foods and alcohol should also be avoided. Once again, the dietician should be involved in the management of patients with mucositis.

Nursing management

Patients with dysphagia should be encouraged to sit upright when eating, preferably in a chair, or well supported in bed if not able to be up. This maintains the normal anatomy and physiology for eating as far as possible. Patients who wear dentures should be encouraged to put them in before eating and they should be kept clean before and after. The patient's nutritional requirements need to be assessed by the dietician and followed as far as possible by nursing staff. The patient should be encouraged to take small amounts and to chew them properly and slowly. The patient should be told to swallow one mouthful at a time before starting another. Fluids are important to moisten food and should be within the patient's reach and of a type the patient likes. Encouraging the patient to drink water, milk or juice with the meal followed by tea or coffee later will help to prevent pain or indigestion in mucositis or candida infection.

Bowel obstruction

Intestinal obstruction is particularly common in ovarian cancer and colorectal cancer; it is also seen less commonly in cancer of the pancreas, stomach, bladder, endometrium and prostate. Obstruction can be caused by either the tumour mass itself (65% of patients), the treatment, e.g. adhesions (25%), or a new tumour (10%) (Waller and Caroline, 2000).

Pathophysiology

Intestinal obstruction leads to an accumulation of fluid, gas, saliva, and gastric and biliary contents. This causes distension, which in turn leads to oedema, congestion, necrosis and perforation or rupture of the lumen.

Diagnosis

The first symptom of intestinal obstruction is usually pain, which tends to come in spasms and is often described as 'colicky'. Patients may report passing blood and mucus rectally, but no faeces or flatus. Vomiting is common. At first it is usually stomach contents, later it is bile-stained fluid from the duodenum and then later it becomes 'faecal', originating from the ileum.

Patients quickly become dehydrated, losing water, sodium and chlorides from the circulation. The patient becomes extremely thirsty, tired and drowsy. Abdominal distension is present with tachycardia, low blood pressure and temperature. The patient will eventually become shocked and if not treated may die.

Patients should have an abdominal X-ray, which will show the dilated loops of bowel.

Management

A nasogastric tube is usually advised to drain fluid, decompress the stomach and relieve nausea and vomiting. The patient is started on an intravenous infusion to replace lost salts and fluids.

Pain control is important and is usually achieved with administration of morphine or diamorphine, by injection.

Obstructions may resolve spontaneously with these measures (conservative management). However, surgical opinions are usually sought and will often lead to surgical intervention. This is usually a resection of the affected part of the bowel with end-to-end anastomosis, a bypass of the affected area with a colostomy or ileostomy or in some inoperable cases percutaneous gastrostomy of the bowel contents.

Diarrhoea and constipation

Diarrhoea

Diarrhoea can be defined as the passing of more than three to four loose or fluid stools in a 24-hour period. Diarrhoea is less common in cancer than constipation (Levy, 1991). Diarrhoea can adversely affect a patient's quality of life and if left can be extremely distressing. Patients often become housebound for fear of soiling and incontinence.

Pathophysiology

The small intestine normally deals with 7–9 litres in a day. This is made up of the oral intake, saliva, stomach contents, pancreatic and biliary secretions. The normal small intestine absorbs 75% of this fluid. The colon then absorbs 90% of the fluid passing through it. As well as fluid, sodium, sodium chloride and glucose are absorbed from the gut.

Diarrhoea means that as well as water, these vital salts and sugars are lost from the system, leading to dehydration and malnutrition.

Causes of diarrhoea in cancer

General debility, fatigue, old age and opioids are major factors in causing faecal impaction. Patients usually experience diarrhoea (overflow) then no bowel movement for several days. On examination the patient often has an impacted rectum, but the rectum may be empty if the impaction is higher in the colon.

Patients with tumours of the colon and ovary are at risk of malignant obstruction either in the lumen of the bowel or without the lumen causing pressure.

The other main causes of diarrhoea in cancer patients are the treatments employed. Radiation enteritis comes on the second week of treatment and lasts 2–3 weeks post-treatments. It is due to damage and sloughing of the bowel lining from the radiation. Chemotherapy, especially 5-fluorouracil for colon cancer, produces diarrhoea as a side effect of treatment. Gastrectomy, ileostomy and total colectomy also lead to diarrhoea as the normal gut physiology is disrupted.

Management of diarrhoea

Patients taking laxatives should stop taking them until diarrhoea stops. If they are taking opiates, e.g. morphine (MST), then the dose of laxatives should be reduced and restarted to prevent constipation becoming the next problem.

Radiation enteritis should be less common with careful planning and small treatment fields (see Chapter 1). Patients are encouraged to avoid fried or highly seasoned foods, uncooked fruit or vegetables and foods, which will cause gas. Oral Sucralfate (1 g, six times a day) has been shown to prevent radiation damage by protecting the mucosa from stool and bile acid irritants (Henrickson et al, 1992).

Diarrhoea caused by chemotherapy cannot usually be prevented and is commonly managed with anti-diarrhoeal drugs. Loperamide hydrochloride (4–8 mg) daily in divided doses, up to a maximum of 16 mg a day, is the usual drug of choice in oncology.

Nursing measures include patient education on correct use of medication, avoidance of possible causes and use of protective pads, pants etc. Patients should be referred to the dietician for advice on foods to help the diarrhoea and those to avoid. The physiotherapist can help with teaching muscle exercises to improve sphincter tone.

Constipation

Constipation is more common in cancer patients than is diarrhoea. A definition of constipation is the inability to expel stool or a decrease in usual frequency (Castle, 1989). The most common cause in cancer patients is the prescription of opioids without adequate laxative cover. Other drugs such as ondansetron or iron can also cause constipation.

Side effects of the disease itself such as debility, fatigue, weakness all lead to a general slowing down of the gut, which causes constipation.

Hospitalisation, having to use commodes or bed pans, lack of privacy all lead to an inability to defecate normally. Bowel obstruction and spinal cord compression are also possible causes.

Management of constipation

Constipation is a common problem and prophylaxis of constipation is a major factor. Patients should be encouraged to be as active as possible physically. Inactivity is a major factor in causing reduced peristalsis and so constipation. Adequate fluid intake of at least 2 litres a day should be the goal as this not only helps to maintain bowel activity but also prevents bladder problems and urinary infections. The constipating effects of drugs such as morphine should be emphasised to patients and any laxatives prescribed prophylactically should be encouraged.

Laxatives

Lactulose (Duphalac, Osmolax) Lactulose is commonly prescribed as a prophylactic laxative. It works by increasing osmosis in the colon and stimulates peristalsis. It also prevents the formation and absorption of ammonia in the colon.

Presentation: oral solution 3.35 g/5 ml.

Dose: 15 ml twice a day adjusted to patient's needs.

The patient should be reminded to take at least 2 litres of fluid per day.

Co-danthramer (Codalax, Codolax Forte) Co-danthramer stimulates muscle activity in the colon, increases water content and thus softens and lubricates the content of the distal colon.

Presentation:

Oral suspension (poloxamer '188' 200 mg and danthron 25 mg/5 ml). Strong oral suspension (poloxamer '188' 1000 mg and danthron 75 mg/5 ml):

Dose: 5–10 ml of co-danthramer or 5 ml strong increased according to the patient's demand/requirements.

Oral intake should be encouraged.

Senna (Senokot) Senokot stimulates peristalsis by acting on Auerbach's plexus.

Presentation:
7.5 mg tablets
15 mg/5 ml granules
7.5 mg/5 ml syrup.

Dose: 2–4 tablets or 10–20 ml syrup taken at bedtime.

The patient needs to be encouraged to swallow tablets with plenty of fluid, as they tend to swell on contact with fluid.

Mouth problems

The mucous membranes of the mouth serve as an important protective mechanism. Intact membranes are involved in support, nutrient absorption, secretion of mucus and salts and enzymes. Cell proliferation in the mucous membranes is fast. Cells live for 3–5 days with a turnover of the outer lining every 7–14 days. This means that the mucous membranes are particularly vulnerable to irritation, trauma or damage, especially from cytotoxic chemotherapy or radiotherapy. The result of this is a general inflammation of the mucosa lining known as mucositis.

Oral mucositis is common and a significant problem in patients with cancer. It can be caused directly by a tumour invading the mucosal lining. Squamous cell carcinoma is the most common – about 90% of mouth cancers (Silverman, 1990). As most oral cancers are advanced at the time of diagnosis it is important to remind patients about regular dental checks. It is at these regular checks that oral disease can be detected early.

The biggest cause of mucositis is the treatment modality used in cancer. Chemotherapy has a direct effect on the mucosa. This is due to high proliferation of the oral cells. The whole reason for using chemotherapy is to destroy cells which are constantly reproducing (see Chapter 1). Therefore as well as destroying cancer cells, chemotherapy will destroy normal cells which reproduce quickly. This mucositis can be severe and the risk is highest with antimetabolites (methotrexate, fluorouracil) and DNA-interactive agents (bleomycin, mitomycin).

Radiotherapy is a localised treatment and so the effects are usually seen in X-ray therapy (XRT) to the head and neck, salivary gland or the mouth itself. A generalised inflammatory response develops as a result of XRT. This will vary with each patient and is dependent on treatment site, field size and dose of radiation used. It usually develops 2 weeks into treatment.

Management of mucositis

The first step in the management of mucositis is daily inspection of the mouths of patients on chemotherapy or having radiotherapy to the head and neck. The first sign is a general reddening and swelling in the treatment field or mouth. As treatment progresses, the mucosa becomes exposed, ulcerated and covered in exudate; pain and discomfort are common and can persist for several weeks after treatment has finished. Mucositis can be complicated by the decline in saliva production when the salivary glands are involved in the treatment site. This is called xerostomia and coupled with mucositis can be extremely debilitating. Opportunistic infection with *Candida albicans* is common.

General measures to manage mucositis include regular oral hygiene and use of mouthwashes to remove debris and prevent infection. As a prophylaxis and in mild cases normal saline is an efficient mouthwash solution. In more severe cases sodium bicarbonate solution can help to remove crusts and benzydamine (Difflam) mouthwash, which is a topical non-steroidal anti-inflammatory drug (NSAID), can be used to relieve pain. Special attention needs to be directed at patient dentures, which should be removed and cleaned carefully. If the gums and mouth are too sore for the patient to tolerate dentures, these need to be kept wet and in a regularly changed disinfectant solution. If the patient has xerostomia a proprietary saliva replacement solution such as Oralbalance or Glandosane can be very effective at relieving dryness.

Patients should be advised to avoid hot or spicy foods and liquids, alcohol and smoking. Cold drinks, yoghurts and puddings will help to soothe sore, damaged mucosa.

Drugs are used to manage infection with candida (see section on dysphagia above), prevent pain and reduce inflammation (benzydamine) and clean the mouth (sodium bicarbonate, saline).

Patients with mucositis are at risk of nutritional deficit if they cannot eat or drink properly due to pain and altered taste; therefore early referral to the dietician is indicated.

Mucositis is unpleasant and can have serious complications. Nurses have an important role in detecting, preventing and treating mucositis.

Lymphoedema

Lymphoedema is the accumulation of lymph in the soft tissues due to a disturbance in the normal lymph drainage. It is seen most commonly in women who have had axillary dissection for breast cancer followed by radiotherapy (40% incidence) (Waller and Caroline, 2000). It also seen in those who have had inguinal node involvement and treatment to the bladder, prostate or ovary.

Causes of lymphoedema

The lymph nodes are damaged by surgery or radiotherapy leading to scarring. They might also become blocked by tumour or metastases. This leads to a failure of the normal function of the lymph nodes in draining lymph. As a consequence, the fluid builds up, resulting in swelling and loss of function.

Management of lymphoedema

First of all, a full clinical evaluation of the patient needs to be carried out. The patient's medical history including primary disease and treatment – surgery, node clearance, radiotherapy – needs to be noted. The amount, level of function/dysfunction and present treatment will be evaluated. The limbs should be measured and compared with opposite unaffected limbs. The pulses need to be recorded. The patient should be asked about how they are coping with activities of daily living.

The management of lymphoedema is variable to say the least. The first point to note is that lymphoedema is permanent and needs to be treated, not cured. The first step is to try drug treatment with diuretics to help drain the venous component of fluid accumulation. The most commonly used drug is Frusemide, 40 mg four times a day. If this does not show any significant difference in 2–3 days, Dexamethasone, 8 mg four times a day, can be used to help reduce swelling around the lymph channels and encourage drainage.

Lymphoedema management is particularly noted as requiring a multi-professional approach. It is a time-consuming, long-term problem. Basic treatment involves education, massage, skin care, compression hosiery and exercise.

Treatment needs to be started as soon as possible and the patient needs to be clear that this is a lifelong problem. Patients need to be told about the correct care of the skin on the affected limb. They need to look for any broken areas, redness or fluid leaks. They should be told not to carry anything heavy with the affected limb, not to have blood samples or blood pressures taken, and to avoid heat or cold.

The physiotherapist will be able to carry out massage and manual lymph drainage, but this must only be performed by those trained to do so. The aim of massage is to increase activity in the unaffected lymph vessels. Once it is seen that massage is helping, the patient and family can be taught to carry out the treatment at home.

Compression bandaging and hosiery are often used. A compression sleeve can be applied to a limb that has mild to moderate swelling. However, in limbs that are very swollen or involve the hand or foot, bandaging is required. Once again, compression bandaging and hosiery application needs to be done by those specially trained to do it. The bandaging or hosiery can be worn all day or removed at certain times to allow for massage and skin care.

Skin care involves washing with simple non-perfumed soap and water. The limb is then moisturised with a non-perfumed moisturiser/emollient cream.

The patient should be encouraged to keep the limb elevated whenever possible and especially at night if not wearing a sleeve or bandage. The physiotherapist will normally teach the patient a range of exercises, which fit in with the individual's needs and abilities. The patient should be in contact with the occupational therapist; activities of daily living may be difficult with a large unmanageable limb. The occupational therapist can help with appliances and changes in the home to make life easier.

Dyspnoea

Dyspnoea is difficult or laboured breathing. It is a common symptom in cancer patients, with an estimated 70% experiencing it in the last 6 weeks of life (Heyse-Moore et al, 1991). Dyspnoea is seen most commonly in lung cancer and metastatic spread from the breast, prostate and colorectal cancer. As well as tumour causes, anaemia and muscle weakness as a generalised consequence of cancer can be causal factors. Table 8.2 shows the multiple factors that can cause dyspnoea in cancer patients.

Management of dyspnoea

The first step in the management of dyspnoea is to identify the cause. The speed of onset is a good indicator. Sudden onset of symptoms usually shows up acute causes such as heart failure, pulmonary embolus or pneumothorax. Onset over days can indicate infection, a superior vena cava obstruction, pleural effusion or tracheal compression. Tumour growth and anaemia are the usual causes of dyspnoea developing over a number of weeks.

Table 8.2. Causes of dyspnoea in cancer patients

Cancer
Tumour obstruction of the trachea and/or bronchi
Tumour infiltration of the small airways or lymph
Pleural effusion
Pericardial effusion
Ascites

Cancer treatment
Surgery: pneumothorax; hypostatic pneumonia
Radiotherapy: radiation pneumonitis
Chemotherapy: drug-induced pulmonary toxicity; anaemia; infection

Other medical conditions
Chronic obstructive airways disease
Congestive heart failure
Asthma

Patients presenting with dyspnoea should have a chest X-ray, ECG and blood gas analysis as well as a full medical examination.

Possible treatment methods include radiotherapy if the cause is obstruction caused by tumour in the main bronchus or trachea. Chemotherapy is used to treat lung metastases.

Non-drug measures used commonly in dyspnoeic patients are calming presence, reassurance and education. Oxygen should be given via nasal prongs as these are less 'claustrophobic' than a mask and are less sweaty and generally better tolerated.

Patients benefit from a cool room and a fan is usually welcomed. The physiotherapist can provide education on breathing exercises, massage and relaxation.

The patient will also be seen by the occupational therapist, who will offer advice on modifications to daily living. Such modifications include moving into one level at home, e.g. move a bed downstairs, sit to wash and shave, and help to deal with all the other activities of daily living.

Drug management will include the following:

- *Salbutamol (Aerolin, Ventolin)*, which produces bronchodilation, increasing voluntary muscle strength. In acute dyspnoea it is usually administered by nebuliser at 5 mg three to four times a day. Once the patient is well enough it can be given by a metered aerosol inhaler, which is 100–200 µg (1–2 puffs), again three to four times a day and as required for breathlessness/wheeze.

- *Diazepam (Valium)* – a sedative used to manage anxiety in dyspnoeic patients. The normal dose is 5–10 mg in acute episodes or at night. Maintenance dose is usually 2 mg three times a day, which can be increased to 15–30 mg per day if required.
- *Morphine* – reduces respiratory drive and is useful in relieving dyspnoea. The normal dose in someone not already taking morphine for pain control is 5–6 mg every 4 hours. Patients already taking morphine should have the dose increased by half.

Dyspnoea is obviously a very distressing symptom of advanced cancer. As it is one of the most common symptoms it is likely that most nurses will have to deal with a patient who has it at some time. Prompt management will reassure the patient and greatly improve quality of life.

Ascites and pleural effusion

Ascites

Ascites, sometimes known as peritoneal effusion, is the accumulation of fluid in the peritoneum. It is usually seen in advanced cancer and is an indicator of a poor prognosis. Ascites is seen in many primary cancer sites, including:

- liver;
- stomach;
- ovary;
- uterus;
- testis;
- breast;
- lung.

In the normal individual a small amount of fluid is present in the layers of the peritoneum to prevent the abdominal organs adhering to the abdominal wall. In malignant ascites, tumour metastases can interfere with the lymphatic drainage of this fluid, which accumulates; liver metastases can cause obstruction in the hepatic venous system, again resulting in ascites. Fluid can reach at least 500 ml before the patient becomes symptomatic. These symptoms are a result of pressure on the abdominal organs leading to pain, discomfort and dysfunction.

Patients usually present with a swollen, tense abdomen, weight gain, lack of appetite, indigestion and constipation.

In mild ascites patients usually respond to diuretics, which can clear up to 1 litre per day. Frusemide, 40 mg orally four times a day, or spirono-lactone, 100 mg orally four times a day, are the usual drugs of choice.

In severe ascites causing any of the symptoms noted above, abdominal paracentesis is the usual treatment. Drainage of the fluid will lead to relief of the symptoms but is not without complications. There is a risk of producing hypovolaemia if fluid is drained too quickly and hypokalaemia and hyponatraemia as result of loss of potassium and sodium ions via the fluid (Kehoe, 1991). The normal regime to try and reduce the risks of hypovolaemia is to drain 1 litre of fluid every 2–4 hours up to a maximum of 4 litres. Regnard and Mannix (1989) state that dryness is obtained over six hours. Some units routinely give human albumin 4.5% 500 ml infusion after every 3 litres are drained. However, the Royal Marsden Hospital (UK) recommends that this is only used if the ascitic protein content exceeds 20 g/litre. In some cases bleomycin or cisplatin are instilled post-drainage to delay or prevent malignant effusion (Ostrowski, 1986; Howell, 1988).

Pleural effusion

Pleural effusion is an abnormal accumulation of fluid in the pleural space. Like ascites it is often a sign of advanced disease and occurs most commonly in bronchogenic cancer. It can be as a direct result of inflam-mation of the pleural surface by tumour mass or infiltration of mediasti-nal lymph nodes by metastases.

The main symptoms of pleural effusion are dyspnoea, cough and pleuritic chest pain. In some cases the patient may not have any symp-toms if fluid accumulates slowly. A chest X-ray will confirm the diagnosis of pleural effusion.

Management of pleural effusion involves pleural aspiration to drain the accumulation of the fluid. This is usually indicated to relieve the dysp-noea. Bleomycin can be instilled to help prevent recurrence. Chemother-apy can be used to manage metastatic spread. Fluid tends to re-accumulate between one and four weeks later but as prognosis is poor, aspiration is the treatment of choice.

CHAPTER 9

Specialist Palliative Care

Throughout the previous chapters the authors looked at the palliative care approach – *basic* knowledge and skills that every health professional should possess. However, there comes a point when knowledge and skills are required to provide continuing optimum care to patients. This is where the specialist palliative care team come in. This chapter looks at the concept of hospital support teams, how they are made up and how they can help nurses in acute areas. The need for defined strategies for referral and intervention are discussed, as are the background and insight of hospice care.

Defining specialist palliative care

Specialist palliative care is defined as 'those services with palliative care as their core speciality. Specialist palliative care services are needed by a significant minority of people whose deaths are anticipated and may be provided: directly through specialist services, or indirectly through advice to a patient's present professional advisers/carers' (NCHSPCS, 1995).

Indirect care through advice

By now you should be aware that palliative care is patient-centred, multi-professional, constantly changing and complex. The starting point needs to be the palliative approach followed by the advice and support of the hospital palliative care team (HPCT). The first such team was established in 1976 at St Thomas's Hospital in London as a terminal care support team (Bates et al, 1981). Most people still die in hospital for a number of reasons. Very often patients are admitted to hospital after suffering an acute event during prolonged cancer management; in some cases this event leads on to a terminal stage of illness. Deterioration can happen so rapidly that patients and families do not have time to make 'end of life' decisions and so arrangements for place of death cannot often be made.

It is in such cases of complex problems relating to symptom management and discharge/terminal care that the HPCT becomes involved.

The normal set-up for such teams is a consultant in palliative medicine and one or more nurse specialists. In the United Kingdom many of these teams have been funded by the Macmillan organisation and they maintain close links to the local hospice or specialist palliative care team. Very often the consultant will have a joint appointment with 'sessions' split between the hospice and acute setting. Within the acute setting and as part of the HPCT, consultants in palliative medicine act in an advisory role. They are normally accessed by another doctor or one of the specialist nurses. Whenever the HPCT is involved, the referring consultant maintains overall responsibility for care. However, it would be uncommon for any advice about management to be ignored after being asked for. Clinical nurse specialists usually have extensive palliative care or cancer experience. Many are now educated to masters degree level. Their main role is in the assessment of patients' palliative care needs and then giving advice and guidance on symptom control, medication, nursing care and if required transfer or discharge planning.

Another major part of the role of the HPCT is teaching both medical and nursing staff. It is vital that those providing basic palliative care are aware of how to access the team, what the team can-provide and when it needs to be involved. This is particularly important in ensuring that the patient receives optimum care. Although most hospitals and HPCTs will have their own referral criteria and procedures, the following gives a guide as to when it might be appropriate to involve specialist palliative care.

Most of those referred to specialist palliative care have disease that is beyond the stage of cure. It would be sensible to involve the specialist palliative care team for the following:

1. Symptom management – difficult pain problems, unresponsive, nausea or vomiting etc.
2. Patients who need hospice, respite or terminal care.
3. Patients with complex psychosocial problems, home problems or money problems.
4. Support or counselling of patient, family or staff.

5. Advice or teaching of patient, family, staff.
6. Lymphoedema management.

In addition to education, research and audit are important aspects of the team's role. Research is a vital component of any health professional's work/training. Evidence-based care has been an integral part of the modern hospice movement (NCHSPCS, 1995). As well as increasing knowledge and allowing development of best practice, involvement in research is one of the elements defining a specialist palliative care service (Glickman, 1997).

Direct care from specialist palliative care

At some point many palliative care patients will reach a stage where they would be best cared for in a specialist palliative care unit or hospice. Hospice and hospice care are terms used to refer to a philosophy of care rather than a specific building or service (NCHSPCS, 1995). With hospice care the approach is to care for people with incurable disease as a whole person. The control of pain and other symptoms takes precedence over curative treatment. The patient, family and caregivers are very much part of the team, which includes medical, nursing therapy, psychology and volunteer staff.

Hospice care can be provided in specially designated units, either voluntary or NHS, or in the patient's home.

It is generally the case that patients who are deemed to have months or less to live if the disease runs its expected course will be admitted to a hospice (Marrelli, 1999). The majority of patients admitted to a hospice will have cancer, although increasingly, patients with HIV/AIDS, end-stage renal, cardiac and lung disease are also being referred for specialist terminal care.

Specialist palliative care involves multidisciplinary teamwork and the usual team is composed of the following.

• One or more consultants in palliative medicine with the appropriate specialist registrar and junior doctor support.
• Nursing staff with basic knowledge of the philosophy and practice of palliative care. Those of senior staff nurse grade and above should hold a recognised post-registration qualification in palliative care. Senior nurses should be educated to masters level.
• Therapy staff – there should be access to physiotherapists, occupational therapists, dieticians and speech therapists.

- Psychology, social work, counselling and religious and spiritual skills must also be available.
- In most hospices complementary therapies and volunteers play an important part in the team.

As we have already said, the main reason for admission to hospice is for terminal care, when it is impossible or inappropriate for this to take place at home. Many patients can also be admitted for respite care or in some cases rehabilitation. Increasingly more patients are attending day centres. This means that they can stay at home longer and be admitted as out-patients for procedures such as pleural and abdominal paracentesis, symptom assessment and control, and medical consultations. Most day centres also provide access to complementary therapy, massage, chiropody and hair-dressing. It also gives patients the opportunity to meet others and gain support.

A major part of the hospice is bereavement counselling and support. Close co-operation, teamwork and nursing mean that it is easier to provide not only professionally trained bereavement counsellors but also in-house-trained volunteer counsellors. These provide ongoing and often prolonged support to bereaved families, as well as one-to-one counselling, and may set up and run groups, with some centres having specific services for bereaved children.

Hospices and specialist palliative care units also play a part in education and development of palliative care services. Many of the bigger units have specific designated education centres. In particular, the major hospices run by Marie Curie Cancer Care are heavily involved in education. Education in specialist palliative care ranges from study days on specific areas, short courses and degrees through to Master degrees.

CHAPTER 10

Palliative Care Emergencies

In this chapter the authors examine some of the more common palliative care emergencies seen in acute care.

1. Infection and neutropenia.
2. Bleeding.
3. Cardiac tamponade.
4. Stridor.
5. Superior vena cava obstruction.
6. Spinal cord compression.
7. Pulmonary embolism.
8. Hypercalcaemia and other electrolyte imbalances.

Infection and neutropenia

Infection is a big problem in the patient with cancer. It has been suggested that it is implicated in at least 50% of deaths in those with solid tumours (Ellerhorst-Ryan, 1993). Patients with cancer are at greater risk of infection due to impaired immune function caused by the disease itself and the side effects of cancer treatment (Peterson, 1998). The risk of infection is related to the level of neutropenia (lowered white cell count). More than 60% of patients with neutropenia will develop an infection (Wujcik, 1999). The majority of these infections will be caused by bacteria. Those that prove fatal are usually caused by a bacterial infection with superimposed fungal infections (Sugar, 1990).

Patients with infection or neutropenia usually need to be admitted to hospital. This has an impact on their quality of life for a number of reasons. They are usually nursed in a side room, visitors are restricted and drugs/antibiotics are usually given by the intravenous route.

Nursing assessment and management

The usual indicator of infection is a raised temperature. Henschel (1985) defines fever as three oral recordings over 38°C in 24 hours or one recording over 38.5°C. Patients having chemotherapy are usually told to record their temperature 4-hourly whilst at home. It is usually at home that their fever is discovered and prompt treatment with antibiotics is recommended.

On admission the patient needs a full assessment, paying particular attention to the patient's recorded temperature over the previous 24 hours. The patient should be asked when they first noticed the fever or chills, stating what action they took, e.g. paracetamol tablets. Any breaks in the skin, tender or red swollen areas should be noted and the medical staff informed. Wound swabs should be taken and sent for culture to identify specific bacteria involved in the inflammatory process. If the patient has a central venous catheter *in situ* for chemotherapy administration, the exit site needs to be examined for redness, exudate or pain. If any of these are present, the site needs to be swabbed.

The patient's temperature, pulse and blood pressure need to be recorded 4-hourly. Comfort measures such as change of clothing or bed linen if wet, fanning and tepid sponging should be implemented as and when required.

Medical management

The patient will be seen by a doctor who will carry out a full physical examination and usually admit the patient to hospital. Specimens of blood, urine and stool will normally be requested and sent for culture. A chest X-ray will normally also be done, to identify a chest infection as the cause.

Patients will normally be given intravenous antibiotic therapy, usually with penicillin to start with until the exact cause is identified.

Patients who are identified and treated promptly usually respond quickly to treatment and support. Precautions such as avoiding crowded places and people with coughs and colds should be encouraged and the patient reminded to record their temperature 4-hourly on discharge. The patient needs to be reminded to carry out these precautions even after chemotherapy course has been completed.

It should be noted that infection is also a natural occurrence in the dying process and that antibiotic therapy usually does not play any part in reversing this case.

Bleeding

There are a number of possible causes of bleeding in patients with cancer. In this chapter we will look at haematemesis and haemoptysis, as these are two of the most common reasons for patients being admitted to hospital.

Haematemesis

Haematemesis or vomiting blood is a common emergency in patients with oesophageal or stomach cancer. The majority of bleeds are slow and usually the result of peptic ulceration from the stress of the disease or a result of drug management, e.g. non-steroidal anti-inflammatory drugs. Massive bleeding is uncommon and usually signifies oesophageal rupture or perforation of liver metastases. These bleeds are usually fatal.

Nursing assessment of haematemesis includes noting the amount and nature of bleeding: whether the bleeding is frank, and just blood that is fresh; whether it is altered, i.e. has been in the gut (usually dark and foul smelling); or is black, indicating a bleed lower in the gastrointestinal tract.

Recordings of the patient's pulse and blood pressure need to be made 2–4-hourly or as the condition changes. The patient also needs to be observed closely for signs of impending shock, e.g. general status, colour, level of consciousness.

The decision to replace blood loss lies with the medical staff, and the nursing staff need to be aware of the procedures and dangers of blood transfusion. Accurate fluid balance needs to be maintained with close attention to urine output.

Haematemesis is usually investigated by oesophagoscopy and gastroscopy. Once the cause has been identified. appropriate treatment can be instigated. Peptic ulceration is usually managed with drugs, e.g. ranitidine or omeprazole in the first instance. Oesophageal varices can be dealt with by sclerotherapy.

Surgical intervention is usually only considered in cases that do not respond to medical management.

Haematemesis is a frightening experience not only for the patient, but also for those who are close to the patient, and the family need careful explanations about the cause of bleeding and the proposed management plan. Close reassurance and attention from nursing staff can help immensely.

Haemoptysis

Haemoptysis is the coughing up of blood and is usually related to bronchial and lung cancer. There are varying degrees of haemoptysis ranging from blood-stained sputum to massive bleeding of 400–600 ml per day. The haemoptysis is usually caused by inflammation or erosion and necrosis of lung tissue or blood vessels or tumour.

Assessment of haemoptysis

Nursing assessment should include noting the nature of the bleeding: fresh blood usually indicates bleeding from the nose or pharynx, but might be from the lower airways: blood from the lungs is more likely be dark coloured. The amount of blood is also very important in helping medical staff decide on treatment. The nature of the sputum is also very relevant; e.g. blood-streaked purulent sputum usually indicates chest infection or if associated with pleuritic chest pain is suggestive of pulmonary embolus (Twycross, 1997).

Management of haemoptysis

Management depends on the cause. Steroids will very often help to reduce mild haemoptysis. The usual drug is dexamethasone, 2–4 mg daily; the anti-fibrinolytic drug tranexamic acid, 1 g three times a day, can also be used with ethamsylate, 500 mg four times a day; this is a haemostatic medication. In prolonged or protracted haemoptysis the patient may be referred for radiotherapy, cryotherapy or laser therapy.

From a nursing perspective the main points of care in haemoptysis are in the support and reassurance of the patient and those around. One needs to inform the patient that fatal haemoptysis is very rare. However, nurses need to be aware that fatal haemoptysis occurs in about 1% of cases (Jones and Davies, 1990). Death is usually due to asphyxia and not haemorrhage (Twycross, 1997).

Cardiac tamponade

Cardiac tamponade results from malignant pericardial effusion (an accumulation of fluid in the pericardium). The causes are usually infection, radiotherapy-induced pericarditis and malignancy (Dragonette, 1998). The usual causes of malignant pericardial effusion are metastases from breast or lung primary tumours. Primary tumours of the heart are rare. Cardiac tamponade occurs when the amount of fluid starts to compress the heart, thus reducing the cardiac output. Cardiac tamponade occurs in 10–30% of patients with cardiac malignancy (Maxwell, 1993). Malignant pericardial effusion carries a poor prognosis.

Management of pericardial effusion/tamponade

The aim of treatment is to remove the accumulated fluid from the pericardium. Before treatment is carried out the patient's stage of disease, prognosis and quality of life needs to be assessed/considered. The usual treatment is pericardiocentesis – drainage of the fluid. This is successful in 94–97% of cases (Vaitkus et al, 1994). Radiotherapy is particularly successful in leukaemia or lymphoma, but breast and lung metastases also respond to this treatment method.

Chemotherapy can be used after pericardiocentesis to help prevent recurrence.

Nursing management

The main aspects of nursing care in this emergency are in patient support. Patients need reassurance and psychological support, both in acute stages and after treatment.

Accurate fluid balance during the administration of blood and fluids is vital to prevent the development of cardiac failure. The patient requires close observation of their vital signs including cardiac monitoring and pulse oximetry. The patient is nursed on bed rest with all the attendant complications; therefore they will need help with activities of daily living.

Pericardial effusion is normally a late sign of malignancy but can be the first sign of cancer. Management is based on many factors including age, primary disease, metastases and prognosis. Nurses need to be aware of all of the factors involved, the management and possible outcomes. Although rare this emergency can occur and so needs to be thought about.

Stridor

Stridor is noisy obstructed breathing caused by airway obstruction in the upper airways and the large main airways. In cancer patients, stridor can be caused by either infection, tumour or metastases.

Stridor caused by infection will usually respond to antibiotic therapy and in the patient with advanced cancer it is usually given by intravenous injection.

Radiotherapy is the normal mode of treatment for stridor due to tumour or metastases. Radiotherapy reduces tumour bulk and so opens the blocked airway. Nursing assessment and management of stridor are similar to those in the breathless patient (see Chapter 8).

Superior vena cava obstruction

Superior vena cava obstruction is usually caused by tumour obstruction to blood flow leading to venous congestion, reduced cardiac output and hypoxia (Morse et al, 1985).The most common non-malignant cause of superior vena obstruction is thrombus.

The obstruction can arise from primary tumour, e.g. small cell or squamous cell lung cancer, or lymphoma, or from metastases from breast or oesophageal tumours.

The presenting symptoms of superior vena cava obstruction are breathlessness caused by the reduced venous return, dilated neck veins and oedematous face, neck and arms. Some patients also complain of headache due to cerebral congestion. These symptoms usually present as an acute emergency.

The usual treatment of superior vena obstruction is a single dose of external beam radiotherapy and a course of dexamethasone. Both reduce the swelling and relieve obstruction.

Nursing care includes assessing and recording the vital signs and oxygen saturation levels. Accurate fluid balance will detect fluid overload, which may necessitate the use of diuretics. Patients invariably need close support and explanations, with the usual precautions in those needing oxygen therapy, i.e. no smoking or naked flames, correct fitting mask, appropriate mask, oral hygiene and oral fluids.

The majority of patients with superior vena cava obstruction respond well to treatment.

Spinal cord compression

This is an emergency which can occur as part of progression of cancer, resulting in partial or total loss of function, either sensory or motor. Cord compression occurs most commonly in tumours of the lung, breast and prostate but can also be associated with lymphoma, renal and head and neck tumours. The compression can occur at various levels: thoracic 70%, lumber 20% and cervical 10% (Kramer, 1992). Dyck (1991) describes spinal cord compression thus: 'The pathophysiological response to spinal cord compression includes oedema of the spinal cord, diminished blood supply at the cord and mechanical distortion of the neural tissue leading to paresis and paralysis.'

Prompt recognition and management of spinal cord compression can help to prevent further damage. The main presenting signs are pain, weakness, sensory disturbance and loss of function.

Diagnosis is based on the patient history and examination, X-ray and MRI scan. Prognosis depends on the level of cord involvement and degree of damage already sustained. Those who have a good function normally maintain this, whereas those with paraplegia have a poor prognosis.

The main treatment for spinal cord compression is steroids and radiotherapy, normally concurrently. The steroids will help pain by reducing the cord oedema whilst radiotherapy reduces tumour bulk.

Nursing management is aimed at preserving motor function and preventing further damage to the spinal cord. Patients need to have anti-embolism stockings applied and are usually prescribed dalteparin (Fragmin) or heparin (Minihep) by subcutaneous injection. Patients are nursed on bed rest and depending on the level of compression may be allowed up to sit/toilet or be completely mobile. Patients need to be observed for signs of chest infection, and temperature, pulse, respirations and blood pressure should be recorded at least 4-hourly. Patients may require catheterisation and accurate fluid balance should be maintained. Blood sugar levels should be checked daily whilst on high dose steroids.

Patients need to have their fears allayed and nurses should be truthful about the prognosis and future.

Pulmonary embolism (PE)

Approximately 10% of cancer patients will suffer a pulmonary embolism (Woodruff, 1999). A pulmonary embolism is the end result of thrombosis from the distal veins in the legs lodging in the pulmonary circulation. This leads to ischaemia and eventually necrosis of the lung tissue. Patients can have multiple small emboli which produce breathlessness, haemoptysis and changes seen on perfusion lung scan. Larger clots produce severe breathlessness, haemoptysis, collapse and hypotension. PE is often implicated in sudden death in those with terminal illness.

Patients with the symptoms described above can usually be suspected of having a PE. In most cases a ventilation/perfusion scan will confirm the diagnosis.

Management

Management will be dependent on severity of the embolism and the condition and prognosis of the patient.

Most nurses are aware that prevention in this case is better than cure. Patients should be encouraged to be as mobile as possible. It is important to ensure adequate fluid intake, and anti-embolism stockings should be used in those at particular risk. In patients with a favourable prognosis and good quality of life, therapy is heparin for 2–3 days and then warfarin for at least 3 months. In those with a history of peptic ulcer or a history of bleeding, anticoagulation will often be ruled out.

In those who suffer massive PE, management is supportive. High flow (10–15 l/min) oxygen, diamorphine to relieve dyspnoea and pain, and psychological support should be given.

Hypercalcaemia and electrolyte imbalances

Hypercalcaemia

Hypercalcaemia (raised blood calcium level) is the most common oncology emergency. It is usually a late complication of cancer and is mostly associated with breast, lung, multiple myeloma, squamous cell cancer of the head and neck and thyroid. The cause is bone resorption from bone metastases and suggests disease progression.

The signs and symptoms of hypercalcaemia include nausea, vomiting, constipation and abdominal pain, tiredness, weakness and increased bone pain and very often confusion.

Treatment of hypercalcaemia involves rehydration with intravenous fluids (normal saline), with supplemental potassium and administration of pamidronate (Aredia) 60–90 mg in 500 ml saline over 4 hours.

Hypomagnesaemia

Low blood magnesium levels are due to poor intake or abnormal loss of magnesium. The disorder causes muscle weakness, confusion and drowsiness. Usual management is intravenous magnesium sulphate.

Hyponatraemia

Low blood sodium levels occur from a number of different causes. Hyponatraemia can be a sign of syndrome of inappropriate anti-diuretic hormone secretion (SIADH) – excess secretion of ADH by tumour (small cell lung) leading to reduced excretion of water, hyponatraemia and increased plasma osmolality.

Symptoms include nausea, general weakness and anorexia. Later patients develop headache, lethargy, confusion and agitation.

Treatment involves careful fluid balance, fluid restriction and use of frusemide.

CHAPTER 11
Terminal Care

Efficient and compassionate care of the dying patient and their family is an integral part of good palliative care. Often referred to as terminal care, this is usually seen as the last 48 hours of life. This can be a difficult time for all of those involved, but by following some basic good practices it can be a favourable time. This chapter will give an idea of what terminal care involves and how adopting the palliative approach can help everyone through.

Symptom control during terminal care

Most distressing symptoms during the terminal stage can be controlled using continuous subcutaneous infusion. There is *no* place in terminal care for the use of intermittent intramuscular injections, and this practice is to be discouraged at all times. This is a painful and unnecessary method of administering medication in what are often elderly, frail patients with little or no muscle mass due to the effects of disease. Continuous subcutaneous infusion (CSCI) is the preferred method. It is most common to use the Graseby syringe driver. This is a small battery-operated pump which delivers a set volume of medication continuously over a 24-hour period. Two models are available – the hourly rate MS16A and a 24-hour rate, the MS26.

Care needs to be taken when selecting a device and it should be checked which driver is being used. Most terminal care and hospital units use the MS16A and we will therefore look at some detail in how to set up and use this particular driver.

When using the MS16A, the drug delivery is based on a 24-hour period. This covers the 'life span' stability of most drugs used in symptom control at this stage, and is the easiest way to run the pump. The volume of drug is based on a stroke length in the syringe of 48 mm. Different sizes of syringe can be used to accommodate different volumes of drug, but the length of fluid must always be 48 mm. For example:

- 8 ml in a 10 ml syringe;
- 14 ml in a 20 ml syringe;
- 17 ml in a 30 ml syringe.

By using 48 mm it is easy to calculate the rate at which to set the driver to deliver the drug over a 24-hour period, i.e.:

48 mm ÷ 24 hours = 2 mm per hour

The pump is then set at 02 on the driver, remembering that this is in mm per hour NOT ml per hour.

Once an appropriate sized syringe has been chosen the pump is connected to the patient via a commercially available 'butterfly' cannula and drug infusion administration set. The butterfly cannula should be secured with a clear adhesive dressing to allow for checks on the site to be carried out. The normal sites are the anterior chest wall, anterior abdominal wall, anterior aspect of the thighs and anterior aspect of the upper arms. These sites need to be checked regularly for any redness, swelling or pain, and rotated as and when necessary. Once the infusion is ready the 'Start/Test' button on the pump is depressed until a small orange light is seen flashing on the driver.

Once the infusion has been running for at least 4 hours, the following points should be checked:

1. The medication's effect on symptom control.
2. The infusion site for irritation, swelling or pain.
3. The syringe for precipitation of the drug.
4. That the driver is running at the set rate and indicator light is flashing.

Indications for using a syringe driver

The Graseby syringe driver is indicated in the following circumstances:

- nausea or vomiting;
- intestinal obstruction;
- dysphagia;
- drowsy, semi-comatose or comatose patient;
- malabsorption causing poor symptom control.

The following is a rough guide to the more common drugs used in a syringe driver to manage symptoms in terminal care. This is only a rough guide and appropriate local policies should be referred to for up-to-date doses etc.

Pain

The drug of choice is diamorphine due to its increased solubility in water, although morphine and fentanyl can be used in some cases.

Nausea and vomiting

Cyclizine is also an antihistamine; Metoclopramide has both an anti-emetic and anti-nauseant effect; Methotrimeprazine has both of these properties as well as a sedative effect; and Haloperidol also acts as an anxiolytic. Chlorpromazine, Diazepam or Prochlorperazine should not be used, as they cause skin irritation.

Corticosteroids

The steroid of choice is Dexamethasone, which is anti-inflammatory. But care needs to be taken when mixing it with other drugs as it can precipitate.

Most of these drugs can be given in combination and will remain stable for up to 24 hours. However, always check that they are compatible and look for precipitation in the syringe. If this occurs, the infusion needs to be stopped and the site changed.

Signs of impending death

As any life-threatening disease progresses there are physiological changes which take place, e.g. increasing hypoxia, respiratory acidosis, altered brain function and renal failure (Berrie and Griffie, 2001). It is generally accepted that death can be expected when the patient starts to experience the following signs and symptoms (NCHSPCS, 1997b; Twycross and Lichter, 1998):

- profound weakness – patient is unable to perform any activities of living unaided;
- gaunt and pale appearance;
- loss of interest in surroundings, extensive periods of drowsiness and sometimes disorientation;

- no wish to eat or drink;
- inability to swallow medications etc.

It is imperative that the patient's family are aware of the significance of these signs and that they are kept up to date with what the professional carers are thinking. This can be a problem in acute areas, where despite all efforts at cure, the patient is clearly not getting any better, or their symptoms are getting worse. Medical staff may continue to strive towards cure, overlooking the patient's quality of life. Sudden cardiac arrest as an acute event is relatively uncommon in patients with advanced cancer, yet such a dramatic event remains uppermost in the thoughts of many health care professionals. It is of course relevant to be aware of both patient and families wishes in relation to cardiopulmonary resuscitation, but one must always be aware that the majority of patients will die quite calmly and peacefully – if we can adopt the palliative approach.

Nursing care

It is natural at this stage of the cancer journey for relatives to want to stay with the patient, and this should be accommodated. If possible the patient should be nursed in a single room to provide privacy, not only for the family, but for the other patients who may have to cope with the impending death.

The family and nurses should be encouraged to speak to the patient and hold normal conversations whilst in the room or carrying out care. This is especially important whilst the patient remains lucid. Nurses must maintain normal practices of giving explanations of care to both the patient and family. Remember that hearing is the last sense to be lost and be mindful of what is said in the presence of the patient. Reduce unnecessary stimuli to the patient such as bright overhead lights and loud noises from the ward.

The room temperature needs to be adapted to meet the needs of the patient. If they are too hot or too cold then it is the role of the nurse to deal with this. The family can adapt to their own needs, the patient is dependent on the nurse. Also remember that a small room full of people can become quite stuffy and claustrophobic so keep it ventilated and as tidy as possible. Avoid lots of equipment, tables or chairs.

By the time the patient has reached this stage, their need for fluids has naturally reduced; therefore artificial hydration is usually of little benefit. The use of intravenous infusions, nasogastric feeds etc. should be discontinued after an explanation to the family. If medical staff insist on continuing intravenous fluids these should be reduced to 12–24-hourly bags.

The patient's position in bed needs to be changed 2–4-hourly. This not only prevents pressure sores, but helps reduce the build-up of bronchial secretions. The build-up of these secretions in the trachea and larynx causes the symptom often called 'death rattle'. Although this is distressing for those around it is not as bad as people think for the patient. If caught early enough the anticholinergic drug hyoscine can reduce the fluid. However, if it is used late it will have little effect. Suctioning is NOT appropriate as it irritates the mucosal lining and leads to the production of increasing amounts of mucus. If it is necessary it should be restricted to the mouth, throat and nasopharynx.

Whilst changing the patient's position take time to carry out other 'basic' nursing care such as mouth care, eye care if necessary and pressure area checks. If patients are incontinent, change the linen and use pads to protect the sheets. Catheterisation should be avoided in all but extreme cases of incontinence due to the associated problems of infection. Remember that meticulous skin care is necessary whenever the patient is incontinent of either urine or stool.

As death becomes imminent the patient's skin becomes cold and clammy to touch. Often beads of sweat can be seen on the forehead. The extremities become cold and mottled in colour, and the radial pulse is often weak or absent. Cyanosis of the nose, nail beds and knees is evident.

Immediately before death the patient's breathing pattern often changes and they often experience Cheyne–Stokes pattern. Death is often peaceful with breathing stopping followed shortly by the heart.

Time of death

It is usually obvious to all those present that the patient has died. There will be no respiratory effort, central pulses will be absent and the pupils do not respond to light. In many places an experienced registered nurse can verify expected deaths but a registered medical practitioner must still certify that death has occurred. If the family are present at the time of death, the nurse needs to tell them that the patient has actually died. It is often appropriate at this point to leave them with the patient whilst you inform the doctor of the death. However, if the relative is elderly or alone they might wish you to stay with them at this time and you need to gauge their needs on an individual basis.

When the doctor does arrive he needs to carry out an examination of the patient to certify death and this is often a good point to ask the relatives to leave the room for a time. Take them to a private room which is comfortable and quiet. Ward offices are not a good place as the phone often rings, people need access and it is generally not very private. Have a supply of tissues, and the customary cup of tea to hand. If they want privacy give it, if they want you to stay do so.

The doctor will examine the patient and then make an entry in the medical notes. This usually includes the following:

- date and time seen;
- general appearance of the body;
- pupillary reflex – fixed and dilated;
- absent breath and lung sounds;
- absent carotid and apical pulse;
- signature and status;
- RIP.

In cases where the death is expected and the doctor is happy that there is no foul play a death certificate will then be issued to the next of kin. This should be given to the family along with an explanation of the procedures to be followed in registering the death and contacting an undertaker. Most hospitals have information packs and booklets which the family can take away to read later. An excellent reference is Hanna Cooke's book *When Someone Dies* (Cooke, 2000), which gives detailed information on the different procedures to be followed with religious beliefs and faiths. Different hospitals will have local rules regarding patients' belongings and personal effects and these should be followed.

Care of the body

Once the doctor has finished, the family have said their goodbyes and any religious practices have been carried out, it is customary for the nurses to carry out last offices. This should be done as per hospital policy but generally follows a similar pattern.

Ensure that the patient's eyes and mouth are closed. Sometimes the mouth will not close and should be left; avoid putting pillows under the chin or bandaging as these very often do not work. Clean the patient's mouth and replace dentures if they fit. Often the patient has lost so much weight that this is not possible. However, the dentures should be sent with the patient for the attention of the mortuary staff or undertaker. The body should be washed and the hair combed into the patient's usual style. Avoid shaving male patients as you can often nick the skin, and in some cases patients have had beards shaved off that they had for many years whilst alive. This can cause considerable distress to families, so shaving is best left to the undertaker. All wounds should be covered with a water-proof dressing, catheters and drains should be removed and any holes covered. If continual or excess drainage occurs, then the appropriate orifice can be lightly packed with cotton wool. The patient should be dressed in a shroud unless alternative arrangements have been made with the family. The patient needs to be identified with a legible wrist band and a tag attached to the great toe. The body is then wrapped in a sheet secured with adhesive tape and transported in a covered trolley to the mortuary. The body is usually collected by porters and needs to be removed discreetly to avoid distress to other patients or hospital visitors.

Throughout these procedures be mindful of universal precautions to prevent infection. The room needs to be cleaned and ventilated before being used again.

Staff support

Many of the deaths we see in cancer patients are the culmination of a long hard journey from diagnosis, through treatment to death. The patient and their family have often become very close to those caring for them. We all need to be aware of our own and others' feelings surrounding the death of any patient. Remember that everyone in the ward can be affected and that peer support is essential in coping with such an event.

References

American Nursing Association (1991) Task force on the nurse's role in end of life decisions. American Nursing Association. Position Statements – Nursing and the Patient Self-Determination Act, 1991. Washington DC.

Archer J (1991) The process of grief: A selective review. Journal of Advancement in Health and Nursing Care 1(1): 9–37.

Baines M (1988) Nausea and vomiting in the patient with advanced cancer. Journal of Pain and Symptom Management 3: 81–5.

Barnes K and Barnes M (1991) Effective management of nausea and vomiting. Prescriber October 19: 29–34.

Bates JAV and Nathan PW (1980) TENS for chronic pain. Anaesthesia 35: 817–22.

Bates TD, Hoy AM, Clarke DG and Laird PP (1981) The St Thomas' Hospital Terminal Care Support Team – a new concept of hospice care. Lancet i: 1201–3.

Berrie P and Griffie J (2001) Planning for the actual death. In Ferrel BR and Coyle N (Eds) Textbook of Palliative Nursing. New York: Oxford University Press.

Bonica JJ (1987) Cancer pain: Importance of the problem. In Swerdlaw M and Ventafridda V (Eds) Cancer Pain. Lancaster: MTP Press.

Bowling A (1983) The hospitalisation of death: Should more people die at home? Journal of Medical Ethics 9: 158–61.

British Medical Association (1999) Withholding and Withdrawing Life Prolonging Medical Treatment. London: BMJ Books.

Bruera E and Faisinger RL (1997) When to treat dehydration in a terminally ill patient? Supportive Care in Cancer 5(3): 205–11.

Bruera E, Kuhn N, Miller MJ and Macmillan K (1991) The Edmonton Symptom Assessment System (ESAS) A simple method for the assessment of palliative care patients. Journal of Palliative Care 7(2): 6–9.

Buckman R (1984) Breaking bad news: Why is it so difficult? British Medical Journal 288(1): 1579.

Buckman R (1998) Communication in palliative care: A practical guide. In Doyle D, Hanks GWC and MacDonald N (Eds) Oxford Textbook of Palliative Medicine, 2nd Edition. Oxford: Oxford University Press.

Carter R and Neville A (1988) The aetiology of human cancers. In Tiffany R (Ed.) Oncology for Nurses and Healthcare Professionals, Volume 1, 2nd Edition. London: Harper and Row.

Cartwright A, Hockley L and Anderson JL (1973) Life Before Death. London: Routledge and Paul.

Castle SC (1989) Constipation – endemic in the elderly? Medical Clinics of North America 73: 1497–509.

Cervero F (1991) Mechanism of acute visceral pain. British Medical Journal 47: 549–60.

Chernecky CC and Berger BJ (1998) Advanced and Critical Care Oncology Nursing. Managing Primary Complications. Philadelphia, PA: WB Saunders.

Clegg F (1988) Grief and loss in elderly people in a psychiatric setting. In Chigier E (Ed.) Grief and Mourning in Contemporary Society, Volume 1: Psychodynamics. Freund.

Coates A, Abraham S, Kaye SB, et al (1983) On the receiving end: patient perceptions of the side effects of cancer chemotherapy. European Journal of Cancer and Clinical Oncology 19: 203–8.

Coleman RE and Hancock BW (1996) Cytotoxic chemotherapy: principles and practice. In Hancock BW (Ed.) Cancer Care in the Hospital. Oxford: Radcliffe Medical Press.

Cooke H (2000) When Someone Dies. A Practical Guide to Holistic Care at the End of Life. Oxford: Butterworth Heinemann.

Coursey K, et al (1975) Comparative anxiety levels of cancer patients and family members. Proceedings of the American Association for Cancer Research 16: 246.

Davis DB (2000) Caring for People in Pain. Routledge Essentials for Nurses. London: Routledge.

Doyle D, Hanks GWC and Macdonald N (1998) Oxford Textbook of Palliative Medicine, 2nd Edition. Oxford: Oxford University Press.

Dragonette P (1998) Malignant pericardial effusion and cardiac tamponade. In Chernecky CC and Berger BJ (Eds) Advanced and Critical Care Oncology Nursing. Managing Primary Complications. Philadelphia, PA: WB Saunders.

Dunlop R (1998) Cancer: Palliative Care. Focus on Cancer Series. London: Springer.

Dunlop RJ and Hockley JM (1998) Hospital Based Palliative Care Teams. The Hospital–Hospice Interface, 2nd Edition. Oxford: Oxford University Press.

Dyck S (1991) Surgical instrumentation as a palliative treatment for spinal cord compression. Oncology Nursing Forum 18(3): 515–21.

Ellerhorst-Ryan JM (1993) Infection. In Groenwald SL, Frogge MH and Goodman M (Eds) Cancer Nursing: Principles and Practice. Boston, MA: Jones and Bartlett.

Ellershaw JE, Sutcliffe JM and Saunders CM (1995) Dehydration and the dying patient. Journal of Pain and Symptom Management 10: 192–7.

Ernst E and Fialka V (1994) Ice freezes pain? A review of the clinical effectiveness of analgesic cold therapy. Journal of Pain and Symptom Management 9(1): 56–9.

Fallon M and O'Neill B (1998) ABC of Palliative Care. London: BMJ Publishing Group.

Farber JM et al (1984) Psychosocial distress in oncology outpatients. Journal of Psychosocial Oncology 2: 109–18.

Ferrel-Torry A and Glick O (1993) The use of therapeutic massage as a nursing intervention to modify anxiety and the perception of cancer pain. Cancer Pain 16(2): 93–101.

Finlay I (1995) The management of other frequently encountered symptoms. In Penson J and Fisher R (Eds) Palliative Care for People with Cancer, 2nd Edition. London: Arnold.

Glickman M/Working Party on Standards in Specialist Palliative Care (1997) Making Palliative Care Better: Quality improvement, multiprofessional audit and standards. Occasional paper 12. London: NCHSPCS.

Goyns MH, Hancock BW and Rees RC (1996) Incidence and epidemiology. In Hancock BW (Ed.) Cancer Care in the Hospital. Oxford: Radcliffe Medical Press.

Greer S (1985) Cancer: Psychiatric aspects. In Grossman G (Ed.) Recent Advances in Clinical Psychiatry. Edinburgh: Churchill Livingstone.

Hardcastle JO, Thomas WM, Chamberlain J, et al (1989) Randomised controlled trial of faecal occult blood screening for colorectal cancer. Results of the first 107 349 subjects. Lancet i: 1160–4.

Hawthorn J and Redmond K (1999) Pain: Causes and Management. Oxford: Blackwell Science.

Henrickson R, Franzen L and Littbrand B (1992) Effects of sucralfate on acute and late bowel discomfort following radiotherapy of pelvic cancer. Journal of Clinical Oncology 10: 969–75.

Henschel L (1985) Fever patterns in the neutropenic patient. Cancer Nurse 8: 301–5.

Herd EB (1990) Terminal care. A review of past changes and future trends. Journal of Public Health Medicine 15(1): 3–8.

Heyse-Moore LH, Ross V and Mulee M (1991) How much of a problem is dyspnoea in advanced cancer? Palliative Medicine 5: 27–33.

Higginson I (1997) Palliative and Terminal Care. Health Care Needs Assessment. The Epidemiologically Based Needs Assessment Reviews, 2nd Series. Oxford: Radcliffe Medical Press.

Hockley J, Dunlop R and Davies RJ (1998) Survey of distressing symptoms in dying patients and their families in hospital and the response to a symptom control team. British Medical Journal 296: 1715–17.

Horowitz MJ (1970) Psychological response to serious life events. In Hamilton V and Warburton DM (Eds) Human Stress and Cognition: An Information Processing Approach. Chichester: John Wiley and Sons.

Hoskin P and Makin W (1998) Oncology for Palliative Medicine. Oxford: Oxford University Press.

Howell SB (1998) Intraperitoneal chemotherapy for ovarian cancer. Journal of Clinical Oncology 6: 1673–5.

International Association for the Study of Pain (IASP) (1986) IASP Subcommittee on Taxonomy. Classification of chronic pain. Pain (Supplement 3): 216–21.

International Union Against Cancer (1997) TNM Classification of Malignant Tumours, 5th Edition. New York: Zeneca Oncology.

Jacobs S (1993) Pathologic Grief: Maladaption to Loss. Washington DC: American Psychiatric Press.

James EA (1991) Nursing patients having cancer surgery. In Tiffany R (Ed.) Oncology for Nurses and Healthcare Professionals, Volume 1, 2nd Edition. London: Harper and Row.

Jones DK and Davies RJ (1990) Massive haemoptysis. British Medical Journal 300: 889–90.

Kaye P (1996) Breaking Bad News (Pocket Book). Nottingham: EPL Publications.

Kehoe C (1991) Malignant ascites: etiology, diagnosis and treatment. Oncology Nursing Forum 18: 523–30.

Kendrick K (1998) Bereavement Part 1: Theories of bereavement. Professional Nurse 14(1): 59–62.

Kirby RS, Brawer MK and Denis LJ (1998) Fast Facts – Prostate Cancer, 2nd Edition. Oxford: Health Press.

Kramer JA (1992) Spinal cord compression in malignancy. Palliative Medicine 6: 202–11.

Kubler-Ross E (1970) On Death and Dying (14th Reprint, 1995). London: Routledge.

Lazarus RS and Folkman S (1984) Stress, Appraisal and Coping. New York: Springer Verlag.

Levy MH (1991) Constipation and diarrhoea in cancer patients. Cancer Bulletin 43: 412–22.

Lindbrick E, Elfuing J, Frisell J, et al (1996) Neglected aspects of false positive findings of mammography in breast cancer screening; analysis of false positive cases from the Stockholm Trial. British Medical Journal 312: 273–6.

Lindley CM and Hirsch JD (1992) Nausea and vomiting and cancer patients' quality of life. A discussion of Professor Selby's paper. British Journal of Cancer 66 (Supplement 19): S26–9.

Lorigan PC and Hancock BW (1996) Education, screening, prevention and surveillance. In Hancock BW (Ed.) Cancer Care in the Hospital. Oxford: Radcliffe Medical Press.

Lunt B and Hillier R (1981) Terminal care: Present services and future priorities. British Medical Journal 283: 595–8.

Marrelli TM (1999) Hospice and Palliative Care Handbook. Quality, Compliance and Reimbursement. New York: Mosby.

Martin M (1992) Myths and realities of antiemetic treatment. British Journal of Cancer 19: S46–S50.

Maxwell MB (1993) Malignant effusions and oedemas. In Groenwald SL, Frogge MH and Goodman M (Eds) Cancer Nursing: Principles and Practice. Boston, MA: Jones and Bartlett.

McCaffrey M and Beebe A (1994) Pain: Clinical Manual for Nursing Practice. Adapted from US Edition by Latham J and Bell D. UK Edition. London: Mosby.

McNamarra P (1994) Massage for People with Cancer. London: Wandsworth Cancer Support Centre.

Melzack R and Wall P (1965) Pain mechanisms: A new theory. Science 150: 971–9.

Mobily P, Herr K and Nicholson A (1994) Validation of cutaneous stimulation interventions for pain management. International Journal of Nursing Studies 31(6): 533–44.

Moorey S (1992) The psychological impact of cancer. In Webb P and Tiffany R (Eds) Oncology for Nurses and Health Care Professionals, 2nd Edition. Volume 2: Care and Support. London: Chapman and Hall.

Morse LK, Henry ML and Flynn KT (1985) Early detection to avert the crisis of superior vena cava syndrome. Cancer Nursing 8(4): 228–32.

National Council for Hospice and Specialist Palliative Care Services (1995) Specialist Palliative Care: A Statement of definitions. Occasional Paper 8. October 1995. London: NCHSPCS.

NCHSPCS (National Council for Hospice and Specialist Palliative Care Services) (1995) Specialist Palliative Care – A statement of definitions. Occasional Paper 8. October. London: NCHSPCS.

NCHSPCS (1997a) Feeling Better: Psychosocial Care and Specialist Palliative Care. A Discussion Paper. Occasional Paper 13. August 1997. London: NCHSPCS.

NCHSPCS (1997b) Ethical Decision Making in Palliative Care: Artificial Care for People who are terminally ill. Guidance Paper. London: NCHSPCS.

Neal AJ and Hoskin PJ (1997) Clinical Oncology: Basic Principles and Practice, 2nd Edition. London: Arnold.

Ostrowski M (1986) An assessment of the long-term results of controlling the reaccumulation of malignant effusions using intracavitary bleomycin. Cancer 57: 721–7.

Parkes CM (1972) Bereavement. Studies of Grief in Adult Life. London: Tavistock.

Parkes CM (1988) Bereavement as a psychological transition: Process of adaption to change. Journal of Social Issues 44(3): 53–65.

Parsons T (1992) The social system. In Webb P and Tiffany R (Eds) Oncology for Nurses and Health Care Professionals, 2nd Edition. Volume 2: Care and Support. London: Chapman and Hall.

Pearson A, Vaughan B and Fitzgerald M (1996) Nursing Models for Practice, 2nd Edition. Oxford: Butterworth Heinemann.

Peck A (1972) Emotional reactions to having cancer. American Journal of Roentgenology, Radium Therapy and Nuclear Medicine 14: 591–9.

Peterson PG (1998) Sepsis and septic shock. In Chernecky CC and Berger BJ (Eds) Advanced and Critical Care Oncology Nursing. Managing Primary Complications. Philadelphia, PA: WB Saunders.

Pugsley R and Pardoe J (1992) The sociological impact of cancer. In Webb P and Tiffany R (Eds) Oncology for Nurses and Health Care Professionals, 2nd Edition. Volume 2: Care and Support. London: Chapman and Hall.

Raven RW (1984) The surgeon and oncology. Clinical Oncology 10: 311–18.

Regnard C and Mannix K (1989) Management of ascites in advanced cancer – a flow diagram. Palliative Medicine 4: 45–7.

Ripamonti C, Ticozzi C, Zecca E, Rodriguez CH and De Conno F (1996) Continuous subcutaneous infusion of Ketoralac in cancer neuropathic pain unresponsive to opioid and adjuvant drugs. A case report. Tumori 82: 413–15.

Rosenberg SA (1985) The changing approach to cancer surgery. Hospital Practice 20(3): 105–24.

Silverman S (1990) Oral Cancer, 3rd Edition. Atlanta: American Cancer Society.

Sims S (1986) Slow stroke back massage for cancer patients. Nursing Times 82: 47–50.

Smith SA (1995) Patient induced dehydration: Can it ever be therapeutic. Oncology Nursing Forum 22: 1487–91.

Snape D and Robinson A (1988) Radiotherapy. In Tschudin V (Ed.) Nursing the Patient with Cancer, 2nd Edition. London: Prentice Hall.

Solomon MZ, O'Donnel L, Jennings B, Guilfoy V, et al (1993) Doctors near the end of life: Professional views on life sustaining treatments. American Journal of Public Health 83: 14–27.

Souhami R and Tobias J (1998) Cancer and its Management, 3rd Edition. Oxford: Blackwell Science.

Stedeford A (1981) Couples facing death: Unsatisfactory communication. British Medical Journal ii: 1098.

Stevenson C (1995) Aromatherapy. In Rankin-Box D (Ed.) The Nurses Handbook of Complementary Therapies. Edinburgh: Churchill Livingstone.

Straka DA (1997) Are you listening? Have you heard? Advanced Practice Nursing Quarterly 3(2): 80–1.

Sugar AM (1990) Empiric treatment of fungal infections in the neutropenic: Review of interventions and guidelines for use. Archives of Internal Medicine 150: 2258–64.

Tabar L, Fagerberg G Day NE, Duffy SW and Kitchin RM (1992) Breast cancer treatment and natural history: New insights from results of screening. Lancet 339: 412–14.

Twycross R (1997) Symptom Management in Advanced Cancer, 2nd Edition. Oxford: Radcliffe Medical Press.

Twycross R (1999) Introducing Palliative Care, 3rd Edition. Oxford: Radcliffe Medical Press.

Twycross R and Lichter I (1998) The terminal phase. In Doyle D, Hanks GWC and Macdonald N (Eds) The Oxford Textbook of Palliative Medicine, 2nd Edition. Oxford: Oxford University Press.

Twycross R, Wilcock A and Thorp S (1998) Palliative Care Formulary. Oxford: Radcliffe Medical Press.

Vaitkus PT, Herrman HC and LeWinter MM (1994) Treatment of malignant pericardial effusion. Journal of the American Medical Association (JAMA) 272: 59–64.

Waller A and Caroline NL (2000) Handbook of Palliative Care in Cancer, 2nd Edition. Boston, MA: Butterworth Heinemann.

Wickham R (1999) Nausea and vomiting. In Yarbro CH, Hansen Frogge M and Goodman M (Eds) Cancer Symptom Management, 2nd Edition. Boston, MA: Jones and Bartlett.

Wilkes E (1980) Working Group on Terminal Care. National terminal care policy. Journal of the Royal College of General Practitioners 30: 466–71.

Wilkes E (1984) Dying now. Lancet i: 950–2.

Woodruff R (1999) Palliative Medicine. Symptomatic and Supportive Care for Patients with Advanced Cancer and AIDS, 3rd Edition. Oxford: Oxford University Press.

Worden WJ (1984) Grief Counselling and Grief Therapy. London: Tavistock.

World Health Organisation (1990) WHO Expert Committee. Cancer Pain Relief and Palliative Care. No 804. Geneva. WHO Techical Report Series.

World Health Organisation (1996) Cancer Pain Relief. Geneva: WHO.

Wujcik D (1999) Infection. In Yarbor CH, Frogge MH and Goodman M (Eds) Cancer Symptom Management. 2nd Edition. Boston, MA: Jones and Bartlett.

Yarnold J (1995) Breast Cancer. In Price P and Sikora K (Eds) Treatment of Cancer. London: Chapman and Hall.

Zerwekh J (1997) Do dying patients really need intravenous fluids? American Journal of Nursing 97(3): 26–31.

Appendix

Palliative Care Guidelines

1. Breathlessness
2. Constipation
3. Cough
4. Insomnia
5. Lymphoedema
6. Oral care
7. Nausea and vomiting
8. Pain in cancer
9. Restlessness and confusion
10. Weakness and fatigue

Used with the kind permission of North Glasgow University Hospitals NHS Trust Palliative Care Group.

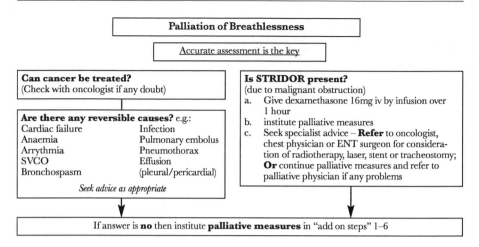

Palliation of Breathlessness

<u>Accurate assessment is the key</u>

Can cancer be treated?
(Check with oncologist if any doubt)

Are there any reversible causes? e.g.:
Cardiac failure   Infection
Anaemia   Pulmonary embolus
Arrythmia   Pneumothorax
SVCO   Effusion
Bronchospasm   (pleural/pericardial)

Seek advice as appropriate

Is STRIDOR present?
(due to malignant obstruction)
a.   Give dexamethasone 16mg iv by infusion over 1 hour
b.   institute palliative measures
c.   Seek specialist advice – **Refer** to oncologist, chest physician or ENT surgeon for consideration of radiotherapy, laser, stent or tracheostomy; **Or** continue palliative measures and refer to palliative physician if any problems

If answer is **no** then institute **palliative measures** in "add on steps" 1–6

---

1.   **Non-drug measures**
•   reassurance, company
•   explanation (patient & carer)
•   stream of air e.g. fan, open window
•   seek advice on positioning – seek physiotherapy input/advice
•   nebulized 0.9% saline 5mls prn helps expectoration but may also help s.o.b.

---

2.   **Consider nebulized bronchodilators**
•   if wheeze/COPD give 2.5-5mg salbutamol nebules qds
•   if still wheezy add ipratropium bromide 0.25–0.5mg nebules qds

---

3.   **Opioids**
•   if opioid naive start with **immediate release oral morphine** 2.5mg 4 hourly and prn. Titrate against symptoms with 30–50% dose increments
•   if can't manage oral start **diamorphine**: 2.5mg bolus subcutaneously prn and set up continuous infusion diamorphine (oral morphine: subcutaneous diamorphine ration = 3mg: 1mg) Titrate against symptom with 30–50% dose increments.

---

4.   **Consider oxygen**
•   certainly if hypoxic (28% via mask or nasal cannulae)
•   can sometimes help even in absence of hypoxia and may be worth a trial but be aware of placebo dependency
•   saturations may be helpful if in hospital and higher concentrations given.

---

5.   **Benzodiazepines**
•   certainly if anxiety
•   often help in absence of overt anxiety (but not a substitute for number 1)

Anxiolytic benzodiazepines

Lorazepam 0.5–1mg sublingual work quickly – may help respiratory panic attack
Diazepam 2–5mg orally and if effective prescribe regularly 2–5mg tds
Midazolam: initial 2.5mg bolus – if effective start with 10mg/24 hours by sc infusion
NB sedation is inappropriate for patient who needs to talk.

---

6.   **Noisy breathing**
•   positing may help
•   if not give hyoscine hydrobromide – prescribe 0.4–0.6mg subcut bolus prn
•   if secretions+++ then give up to 2.4mg via sc syringe driver over 24 hours
•   suction may be required for oropharyngeal secretions – but is not recommended

Constipation in Palliation Care

Common cancer in patients due to general debility, low food and fluid intake, metabolic upset e.g. hypercalcaemia and drug therapy (e.g. anticholinergics, vinca alkaloids and opioids) and central nervous system, lesions e.g. spinal cord compression. Prevention is an important consideration in these conditions.

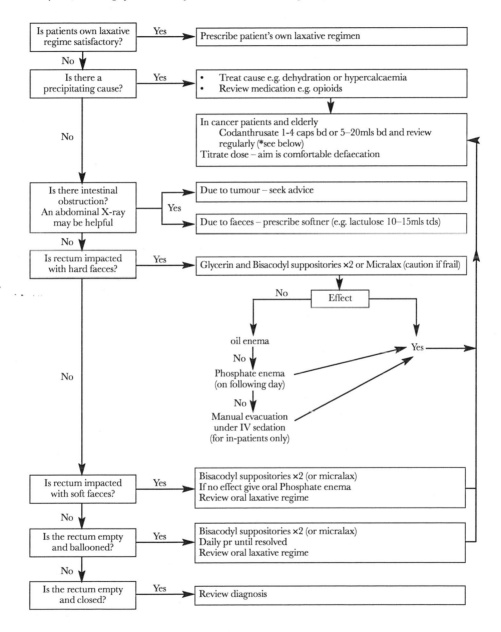

*NB – if faecal incontinence then risk of "danthron burn" – switch to lactulose/senna combination
If patient has stoma and oral laxatives are ineffective – seek advice from stoma care sister

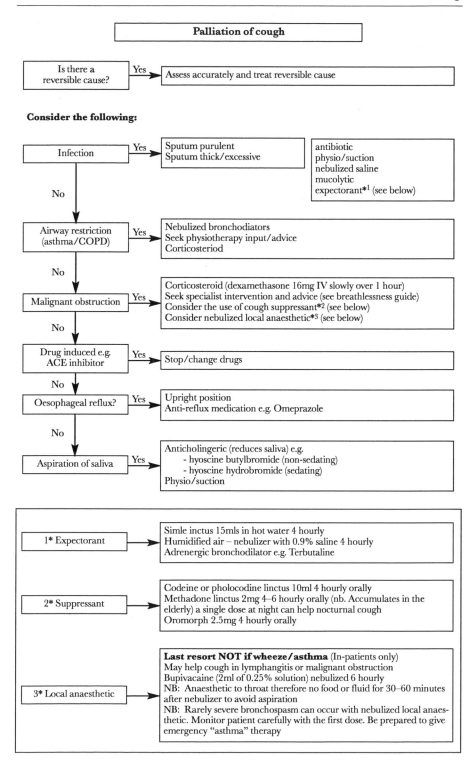

Palliation of cough

| Is there a reversible cause? | Yes → | Assess accurately and treat reversible cause |

Consider the following:

| Infection | Yes → | Sputum purulent
Sputum thick/excessive | antibiotic
physio/suction
nebulized saline
mucolytic
expectorant*¹ (see below) |

No ↓

| Airway restriction (asthma/COPD) | Yes → | Nebulized bronchodiators
Seek physiotherapy input/advice
Corticosteriod |

No ↓

| Malignant obstruction | Yes → | Corticosteroid (dexamethasone 16mg IV slowly over 1 hour)
Seek specialist intervention and advice (see breathlessness guide)
Consider the use of cough suppressant*² (see below)
Consider nebulized local anaesthetic*³ (see below) |

No ↓

| Drug induced e.g. ACE inhibitor | Yes → | Stop/change drugs |

No ↓

| Oesophageal reflux? | Yes → | Upright position
Anti-reflux medication e.g. Omeprazole |

No ↓

| Aspiration of saliva | Yes → | Anticholingeric (reduces saliva) e.g.
 - hyoscine butylbromide (non-sedating)
 - hyoscine hydrobromide (sedating)
Physio/suction |

| 1* Expectorant | → | Simle inctus 15mls in hot water 4 hourly
Humidified air – nebulizer with 0.9% saline 4 hourly
Adrenergic bronchodilator e.g. Terbutaline |

| 2* Suppressant | → | Codeine or pholocodine linctus 10ml 4 hourly orally
Methadone linctus 2mg 4–6 hourly orally (nb. Accumulates in the elderly) a single dose at night can help nocturnal cough
Oromorph 2.5mg 4 hourly orally |

| 3* Local anaesthetic | → | **Last resort NOT if wheeze/asthma** (In-patients only)
May help cough in lymphangitis or malignant obstruction
Bupivacaine (2ml of 0.25% solution) nebulized 6 hourly
NB: Anaesthetic to throat therefore no food or fluid for 30–60 minutes after nebulizer to avoid aspiration
NB: Rarely severe bronchospasm can occur with nebulized local anaesthetic. Monitor patient carefully with the first dose. Be prepared to give emergency "asthma" therapy |

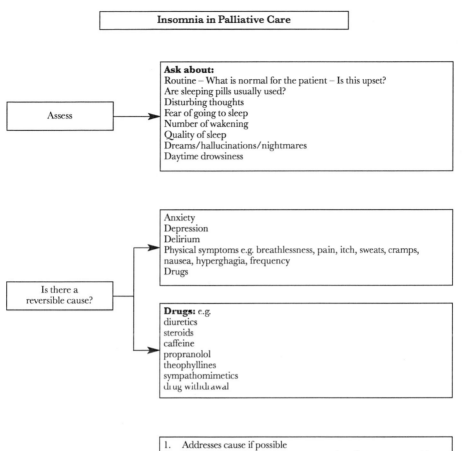

Insomnia in Palliative Care

| Assess | → | **Ask about:**
Routine – What is normal for the patient – Is this upset?
Are sleeping pills usually used?
Disturbing thoughts
Fear of going to sleep
Number of wakening
Quality of sleep
Dreams/hallucinations/nightmares
Daytime drowsiness |

| Is there a reversible cause? | → | Anxiety
Depression
Delirium
Physical symptoms e.g. breathlessness, pain, itch, sweats, cramps, nausea, hyperghagia, frequency
Drugs |
| | → | **Drugs:** e.g.
diuretics
steroids
caffeine
propranolol
theophyllines
sympathomimetics
drug withdrawal |

| Treatment | → | 1. Addresses cause if possible
2. Sleep hygiene plan – promote appropriate sleep pattern; avoid coffee etc.
3. Relaxation techniques – occupational therapy and physiotherapy can help
4. Medication: see below – continue usual medication |

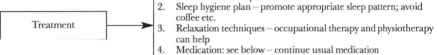

Medication		Dose		Comment
Hypnotic	temazepam	10–40mg	nocte	start low dose
Sedative	haloperidol	0.5–3.0mg	nocte	useful if altered sensorium
	thioridazine	10–50mg	nocte	useful if agitation
Adjuncts	amitriptyline	25–100mg	nocte	sedative antidepressant
	desmopressin	100–300mg	nocte	reduces nocturnal frequency
	quinine	200–300mg	nocte	leg cramps
	baclofen	5–10mg	nocte	leg jerks

5. Lavender (essential oil) – not prescribable but might be recommended to patients e.g. drops on pillow

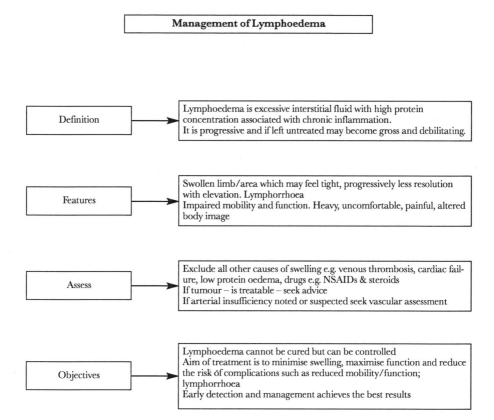

Management of Lymphoedema	
Definition	Lymphoedema is excessive interstitial fluid with high protein concentration associated with chronic inflammation. It is progressive and if left untreated may become gross and debilitating.
Features	Swollen limb/area which may feel tight, progressively less resolution with elevation. Lymphorrhoea Impaired mobility and function. Heavy, uncomfortable, painful, altered body image
Assess	Exclude all other causes of swelling e.g. venous thrombosis, cardiac failure, low protein oedema, drugs e.g. NSAIDs & steroids If tumour – is treatable – seek advice If arterial insufficiency noted or suspected seek vascular assessment
Objectives	Lymphoedema cannot be cured but can be controlled Aim of treatment is to minimise swelling, maximise function and reduce the risk of complications such as reduced mobility/function; lymphorrhoea Early detection and management achieves the best results

Skin care:	– apply moisturiser e.g. diprobase aqueous cream (lanolin free) to skin after washing – inspect skin daily for infection and abrasions – prompt treatment of any wound cover and treat with antiseptic. If limb becomes red or swollen, hot, tender +/– flu like symptoms star antibiotics – use work gloves e.g. when gardening, washing dishes – use sunscreen to prevent burns – use electric razor or depillatory cream on affected area to reduce risk of injury – avoid venepuncture and blood pressure recordings on affected limbs if possible
Massage:	– stimulates lymph flow in the superficial lymph vessels – patients on their carers can be shown to do simple lymphatic drainage – manual lymphatic drainage performed by one trained in lymphoedema management
Compression:	– shaped tubigrip can be used for sift pitting oedema usually on legs – compression garments can be used to control lymphoedema – garments are measured precisely to predetermined pressure; – do not use garments if they cause pain or if any concern regarding arterial supply (seek advice) or if lymphorrheoa (seek advice) or of chest infection present
Exercise:	– exercise is important since it helps fluid to drain – gentle active or passive movements – exercise should be done while wearing elastic support – support heavy limbs while resting. Slings may be helpful when mobile
Follow-up:	– maintenance, monitoring and support

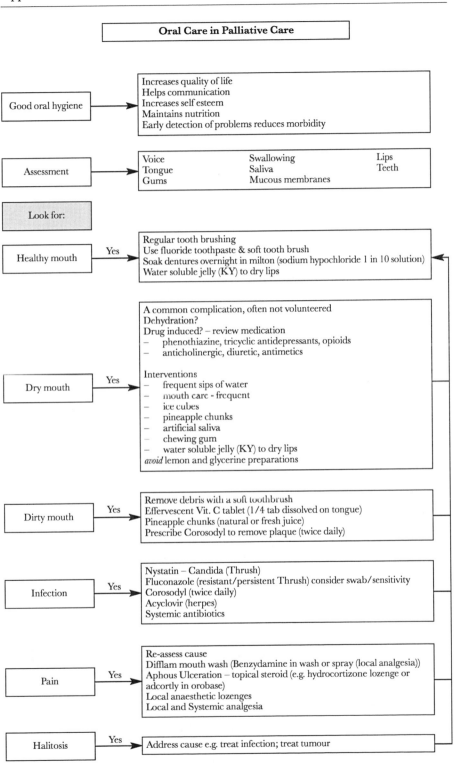

Oral Care in Palliative Care

Good oral hygiene →
Increases quality of life
Helps communication
Increases self esteem
Maintains nutrition
Early detection of problems reduces morbidity

Assessment →
Voice	Swallowing	Lips
Tongue	Saliva	Teeth
Gums	Mucous membranes	

Look for:

Healthy mouth — Yes →
Regular tooth brushing
Use fluoride toothpaste & soft tooth brush
Soak dentures overnight in milton (sodium hypochloride 1 in 10 solution)
Water soluble jelly (KY) to dry lips

Dry mouth — Yes →
A common complication, often not volunteered
Dehydration?
Drug induced? – review medication
- phenothiazine, tricyclic antidepressants, opioids
- anticholinergic, diuretic, antimetics

Interventions
- frequent sips of water
- mouth care - frequent
- ice cubes
- pineapple chunks
- artificial saliva
- chewing gum
- water soluble jelly (KY) to dry lips
avoid lemon and glycerine preparations

Dirty mouth — Yes →
Remove debris with a soft toothbrush
Effervescent Vit. C tablet (1/4 tab dissolved on tongue)
Pineapple chunks (natural or fresh juice)
Prescribe Corosodyl to remove plaque (twice daily)

Infection — Yes →
Nystatin – Candida (Thrush)
Fluconazole (resistant/persistent Thrush) consider swab/sensitivity
Corosodyl (twice daily)
Acyclovir (herpes)
Systemic antibiotics

Pain — Yes →
Re-assess cause
Difflam mouth wash (Benzydamine in wash or spray (local analgesia))
Aphous Ulceration – topical steroid (e.g. hydrocortizone lozenge or
adcortly in orobase)
Local anaesthetic lozenges
Local and Systemic analgesia

Halitosis — Yes →
Address cause e.g. treat infection; treat tumour

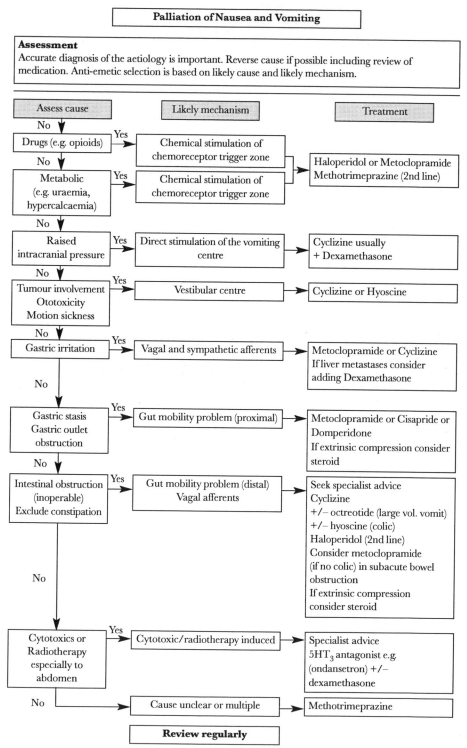

Palliation of Nausea and Vomiting

Assessment
Accurate diagnosis of the aetiology is important. Reverse cause if possible including review of medication. Anti-emetic selection is based on likely cause and likely mechanism.

Assess cause	Likely mechanism	Treatment
No ↓ Drugs (e.g. opioids) — **Yes** →	Chemical stimulation of chemoreceptor trigger zone	
No ↓ Metabolic (e.g. uraemia, hypercalcaemia) — **Yes** →	Chemical stimulation of chemoreceptor trigger zone	Haloperidol or Metoclopramide Methotrimeprazine (2nd line)
No ↓ Raised intracranial pressure — **Yes** →	Direct stimulation of the vomiting centre	Cyclizine usually + Dexamethasone
No ↓ Tumour involvement Ototoxicity Motion sickness — **Yes** →	Vestibular centre	Cyclizine or Hyoscine
No ↓ Gastric irritation — **Yes** →	Vagal and sympathetic afferents	Metoclopramide or Cyclizine If liver metastases consider adding Dexamethasone
No ↓ Gastric stasis Gastric outlet obstruction — **Yes** →	Gut mobility problem (proximal)	Metoclopramide or Cisapride or Domperidone If extrinsic compression consider steroid
No ↓ Intestinal obstruction (inoperable) Exclude constipation — **Yes** →	Gut mobility problem (distal) Vagal afferents	Seek specialist advice Cyclizine +/− octreotide (large vol. vomit) +/− hyoscine (colic) Haloperidol (2nd line) Consider metoclopramide (if no colic) in subacute bowel obstruction If extrinsic compression consider steroid
No ↓ Cytotoxics or Radiotherapy especially to abdomen — **Yes** →	Cytotoxic/radiotherapy induced	Specialist advice 5HT$_3$ antagonist e.g. (ondansetron) +/− dexamethasone
No →	Cause unclear or multiple	Methotrimeprazine

Review regularly

Continued

Doses/Routes

Drug Receptor	Bolus Oral Route	Range/24 hour	Subcutaneous Bolus	Subcutaneous Via Syringe Driver	Other Formulations
Cisapride 5HT$_4$	10mg	30mg			Suppository 50 mg
Cyclizine H$_1$ (and muscarinic)	50mg	100–150mg	50mg/8 hourly	100–150mg/24 hours	
Dexamethasone	8mg	8–16mg		8–16mg/24 hours	Suppository 30 mg
Domperidone D$_2$	10–20mg	40–80mg			
Haloperidol D$_2$	1.5–3mg	5–15mg		5–20mg/24 hours	
Hyoscine hydrobromide muscarinic	0.3mg	0.36mg/8 hourly	0.4–0.8mg/4 hourly	0.6–2.4mg/24 hours	Sublingual / Transdermal patch
Hyoscine butylbromide muscarinic	10–20mg	20–80mg	20mg	80–160mg/24 hours	Less sedating than Hydrobromide
Methotrimeprazine D$_2$ (and H$_1$, 5HT$_3$)	12.5–25mg	25–150mg	6.25mg	12.5–200mg/24 hours	Very sedating at high dose
Metoclopramide D$_2$ (and 5HT$_3$, 5HT$_4$)	10mg	40–120mg	10mg	40–120mg/24 hours	
Octreotide			100–200mcg/8 hourly	300–600mcg/24 hours	
Ondansetreon 5HT$_3$	See oncology protocols				

- Prescribe regularly and PRN
- If continuous nausea OR oral medications failed at 24 hours OR vomiting greater than 3 per 24 hours – convert to subcutaneous administration
- Still poor control – review cause, optimise daily drug dose; consider second line antiemetic; seek specialist advice

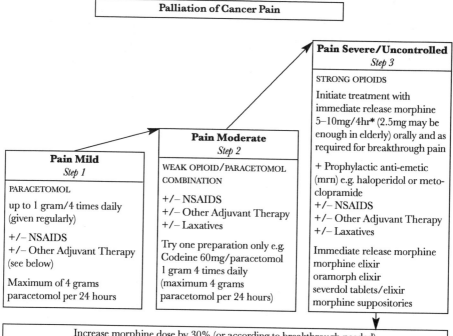

Palliation of Cancer Pain

Pain Severe/Uncontrolled
Step 3

STRONG OPIOIDS

Initiate treatment with immediate release morphine 5–10mg/4hr* (2.5mg may be enough in elderly) orally and as required for breakthrough pain

+ Prophylactic anti-emetic (mrn) e.g. haloperidol or meto-clopramide
+/– NSAIDS
+/– Other Adjuvant Therapy
+/– Laxatives

Immediate release morphine
morphine elixir
oramorph elixir
severdol tablets/elixir
morphine suppositories

Pain Moderate
Step 2

WEAK OPIOID/PARACETOMOL COMBINATION

+/– NSAIDS
+/– Other Adjuvant Therapy
+/– Laxatives

Try one preparation only e.g. Codeine 60mg/paracetomol 1 gram 4 times daily (maximum 4 grams paracetomol per 24 hours)

Pain Mild
Step 1

PARACETOMOL

up to 1 gram/4 times daily (given regularly)

+/– NSAIDS
+/– Other Adjuvant Therapy (see below)

Maximum of 4 grams paracetomol per 24 hours

Increase morphine dose by 30% (or according to breakthrough needed) each day until pain is controlled or side effects intervene

Pain Controlled

Convert to slow release opioid**
a. slow release morphine divide total daily morphine dose by 2 and prescribe 12-hourly (e.g. MST); or once daily morphine (e.g. MXL) may be helpful if patient on too many tablets
b. consider hydromorphone or transdermal fentanyl if slow release morphine inappropriate/problematical (seek advice)

Pain Not Controlled (or side effects intervene)

- Review diagnosis
- Consider adjuvant therapy
- Consider other treatments
- Seek specialist advice

NB *in renal impairment reduce dose +/– frequency
**not advisable in renal impairment – seek advice from pharmacist or palliative care physician

Remember:

Breakthrough Pain Immediate release morphine 1/6th total daily opioid dose (i.e. equivalent to 4 hourly dose) and prescribe as required

Constipation Prescribe appropriate laxatives. Usually stimulant + softener (e.g. codanthrusate or lactulose + senna) and titrate to effect

Explanation for patient and carer

Continue
- Antiemetics prn
- Laxatives
- Immediate release morphine for break-through pain
- Review regularly

Adjuvant Therapy NSAID (e.g. diclofenac 50mg tds) bone, liver, soft tissue infiltration
STEROIDS (e.g. dexamethasone 8–18mg/day) raised intracranial pressure; nerve compression, liver pain
TRICYCLIC ANTIDEPRESSANT (e.g. amitriptyline 25mg nocte – starting dose) nerve pain
ANTICONVULSANT (e.g. sodium valproate 200mg tds) nerve pain
TENS (transcutaneous electrical nerve stimulation)

Parenteral Analgesia (unable to swallow for what ever reason) Parenteral diamorphine dose = 1/3 oral dosage (for equivalent analgesic effect) e.g. patient on MST 60mg bd = 120mg per 24 hrs: divide by 3 = 40mg diamorphine subcutaneous infusion over 24 hrs

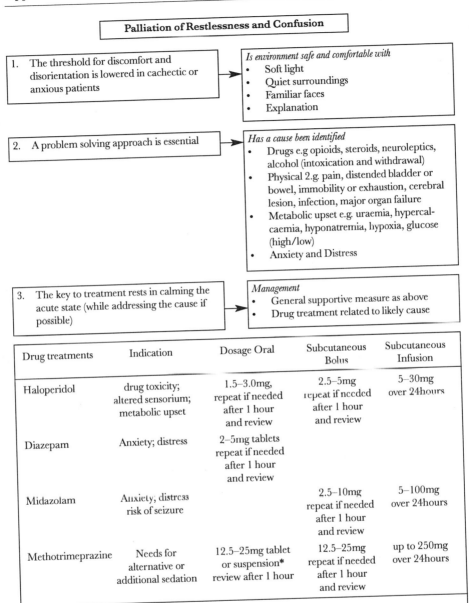

Palliation of Restlessness and Confusion

1. The threshold for discomfort and disorientation is lowered in cachectic or anxious patients

   → *Is environment safe and comfortable with*
   - Soft light
   - Quiet surroundings
   - Familiar faces
   - Explanation

2. A problem solving approach is essential

   → *Has a cause been identified*
   - Drugs e.g opioids, steroids, neuroleptics, alcohol (intoxication and withdrawal)
   - Physical 2.g. pain, distended bladder or bowel, immobility or exhaustion, cerebral lesion, infection, major organ failure
   - Metabolic upset e.g. uraemia, hypercalcaemia, hyponatremia, hypoxia, glucose (high/low)
   - Anxiety and Distress

3. The key to treatment rests in calming the acute state (while addressing the cause if possible)

   → *Management*
   - General supportive measure as above
   - Drug treatment related to likely cause

Drug treatments	Indication	Dosage Oral	Subcutaneous Bolus	Subcutaneous Infusion
Haloperidol	drug toxicity; altered sensorium; metabolic upset	1.5–3.0mg, repeat if needed after 1 hour and review	2.5–5mg repeat if needed after 1 hour and review	5–30mg over 24hours
Diazepam	Anxiety; distress	2–5mg tablets repeat if needed after 1 hour and review		
Midazolam	Anxiety; distress risk of seizure		2.5–10mg repeat if needed after 1 hour and review	5–100mg over 24hours
Methotrimeprazine	Needs for alternative or additional sedation	12.5–25mg tablet or suspension* review after 1 hour	12.5–25mg repeat if needed after 1 hour and review	up to 250mg over 24hours

* needs to be prepared by pharmacy

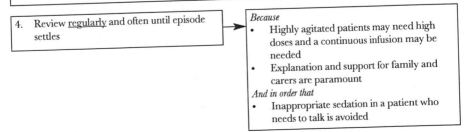

4. Review <u>regularly</u> and often until episode settles

   → *Because*
   - Highly agitated patients may need high doses and a continuous infusion may be needed
   - Explanation and support for family and carers are paramount

   And in order that
   - Inappropriate sedation in a patient who needs to talk is avoided

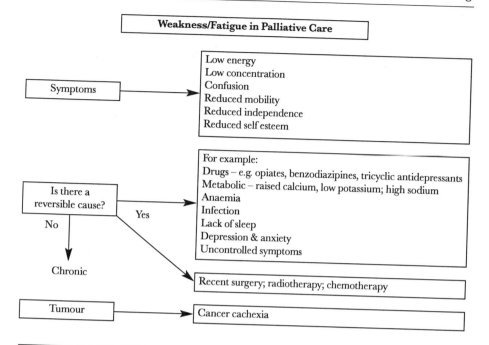

Weakness/Fatigue in Palliative Care	
Symptoms	Low energy Low concentration Confusion Reduced mobility Reduced independence Reduced self esteem

Is there a reversible cause? — Yes →

For example:
Drugs – e.g. opiates, benzodiazipines, tricyclic antidepressants
Metabolic – raised calcium, low potassium; high sodium
Anaemia
Infection
Lack of sleep
Depression & anxiety
Uncontrolled symptoms

No ↓

Chronic

Recent surgery; radiotherapy; chemotherapy

Tumour → Cancer cachexia

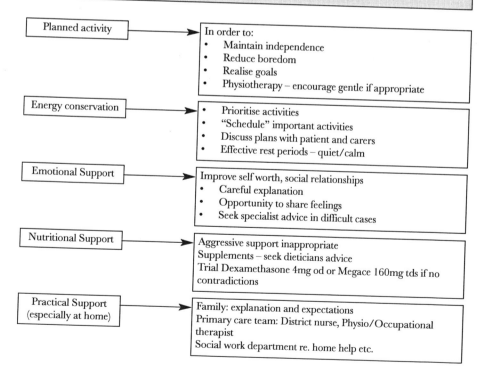

Consider all the following and tailor to individual needs:

Planned activity →
In order to:
• Maintain independence
• Reduce boredom
• Realise goals
• Physiotherapy – encourage gentle if appropriate

Energy conservation →
• Prioritise activities
• "Schedule" important activities
• Discuss plans with patient and carers
• Effective rest periods – quiet/calm

Emotional Support →
Improve self worth, social relationships
• Careful explanation
• Opportunity to share feelings
• Seek specialist advice in difficult cases

Nutritional Support →
Aggressive support inappropriate
Supplements – seek dieticians advice
Trial Dexamethasone 4mg od or Megace 160mg tds if no contradictions

Practical Support (especially at home) →
Family: explanation and expectations
Primary care team: District nurse, Physio/Occupational therapist
Social work department re. home help etc.

Index

acceptance 22
accupressure 54
alkylating agent (cytotoxic) 9
alopecia 10, 18
American Nurses Association (ANA) 26
anaemia 64
anger 21
anticholinergics 54
antihistamines 53
antimetabolites 9
aromatherapy 48
ascites 66, 67
Aspirin 40

bad news, breaking 35
bargaining 21
basic palliative care 13
benzodiazepeines 94
bereavement 16
biomedical Model, of care 11
Bisacodyl suppositories 95
bleomycin 61, 67
blood sample 4
bone metastases 49
bowel obstruction 57, 58, 81
brain metastases 49
breathlessness 94
butyrophenones 53

cancer 1, 13, 15, 16
cancer surgery 6
Candida albicans (Thrush) 55, 56
cardiac tamponade 75, 76
cardio-pulmonary Resuscitation (C.P.R) 28

carcinogens 1
chaplain 29, 33
chemicals 2
chemotherapy (see also cytotoxics) 9, 11, 100
Chlorhexidine mouthwash 56
Cisapride 53
clinical Nurse Specialist 69
Co-danthramer 60
Codiene 40, 44
complementary therapies 47
communication 29, 34–37
constipation 59, 60, 95
coping 17–19, 24, 29
Co-proxamol see Dextropropoxyphene
corticosteroids 54
cough 96
Curie, Marie 7

death 84
'death rattle' 84
denial and isolation 20
depression 21
Dexamethasone 63, 82, 94
Dextropropoxyphene 40, 44
diarrhoea 10, 42, 58, 59
diagnosis and staging 3, 16
Diamorphine 45, 94
Diazepam 66
Diclofenac 42
dietician 32
difflucan see Fluconazole
Dihydrocodiene 44
DNA 7
Domperidone 53

dopamine 52
Do Not Resuscitate (DNR) Orders 28
double Effect 27, 28
dysphagia 54–57
dyspnoea 64–66

electrolyte imbalance 79
epidemiology of cancer 1
essential oils 48
ethical issues 25
euthanasia 29
examination, medical 4

Fluconazole 56
Fluorouracil (5FU) 61
Frusemide 63

general practitioner (G.P) 30
genetics 1
Granisetron 52
guilt 23

haematemesis 74
haemoptysis 74, 75
health education 3
heat and cold application 47
hope 24
hospice 11, 12, 71
hospital palliative care team (HPCT) 12, 68–70
hormones 2
hydration, artificial 26, 27
hypercalcaemia 79
hypomagnesaemia 79
hyponatraemia 79
Hyoscine butylbromide 54

Ibuprofen 43
insomnia 97
International Association for the Study of Pain (IASP) 38
intramuscular injections 80
intravenous infusions 26

Kubler-Ross, Elisabeth 17, 19, 22

Lactulose 60
listening skills 34
Loperamide 59
loss 16

lymph nodes 63
lymphoedema 62–64, 70, 98

Macmillan Nurses 31
massage 46
medical social worker 33
Methadone 96
Metoclopramide 53
Methotrimeprazine 53, 82, 100
Mitomycin 61
models of loss 19, 22
Morphine 40, 45, 66, 94
mouth problems 9, 15, 50, 61, 62
Mucaine 56
mucositis 56, 61
Murray-Parkes, Colin 19, 22

National Council for Hospice and Specialist Palliative Care Services 13, 15, 68
Naproxen 43
nausea and vomiting 9, 27, 50–54, 100
nephrotoxicity 10
neuropathic pain 39
neutropenia 72, 73
non-steroidal anti-inflammatory drugs (NSAIDS) 42
Nozinan see Methotrimeprazine
nuclear medicine 4
nurses 31
nutrition 26

occupational therapist 32
oncology 4, 13, 17
Ondansetron 53, 101
opioids 27, 41, 43
oral hygiene 99

pain 13, 15, 38–50, 102
palliative medicine 30
Paracetamol 40, 41, 42
peripheral neuropathy 10
pharmacist 33
phenothiazines 53
physiotherapist 31, 47, 63
pleural effusion 64, 67
primary appraisal 18
prokinetic drugs 53
psychological care 14, 15, 17, 26
pulmonary embolism 4, 78

quality of life 13,66

radical treatment 5
radiation 2, 49
radiology 4, 8
radiotherapy 7, 8, 9, 48
raised intracranial pressure 51
refusal of treatment 25
restlessness and confusion 103

Salbutamol 65, 94
Saunders, Dame Cicely 12
screening , cancer 2, 3
secondary appraisal 18
Senna 60
serotonin 53
sick role 19
shock 23
specialist palliative care 13, 31
spinal cord compression 60, 77
spirituality 11, 13
stridor 76
Strontium (SR89) 49

suctioning 84
Sucralfate 59
superior vena cava obstruction 79, 94
symptom control 14, 15, 51–67
syringe driver 49, 80

teamwork 14, 35
TENS 48
terminal care 12, 14, 22, 80–86
tissue biopsy 4
TNM system 5
total pain 39
treatment of cancer 5

viruses 2

weakness and fatigue 104
World Health Organization (WHO) 12, 13,
   39

X-ray *see* radiology

Zofran *see* Ondansetron

Palliative Cancer Care in Acute Nursing

Dedication

This book is dedicated to Davina B. Miller (1904–2000), in the sincere hope that no one else suffers as she did in her last days.

Palliative Cancer Care in Acute Nursing

GEORGE HOGG BN, RGN, DipN

Senior Staff Nurse, Tayside University Hospitals NHS Trust, Dundee, Scotland

AND

PAUL CHRISTIE RGN

Staff Nurse, Tayside University Hospitals NHS Trust, Dundee, Scotland

W

WHURR PUBLISHERS
LONDON AND PHILADELPHIA

© 2002 Whurr Publishers
First published 2002 by
Whurr Publishers Ltd
19b Compton Terrace, London N1 2UN, England and
325 Chestnut Street, Philadelphia PA 19106, USA

Reprinted 2003 and 2005

British Library Cataloguing in Publication Data
A catalogue record for this book is available from the British
Library.

ISBN: 1 86156 262 4

Printed and bound in the UK by Athenaeum Press Ltd,
Gateshead, Tyne & Wear